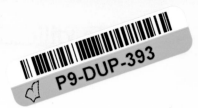

The grammatical analysis of language disability

A procedure for assessment and remediation

David Crystal, Paul Fletcher and Michael Garman

Department of Linguistic Science, University of Reading

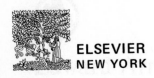

ELSEVIER
NEW YORK

© David Crystal, Paul Fletcher and Michael Garman 1976

First published 1976 by
Edward Arnold (Publishers) Ltd
25 Hill Street, London W1X 8LL

Cloth edition ISBN: 0 7131 5842 5
Paper edition ISBN: 0 7131 5843 3

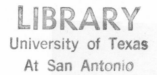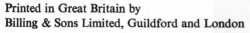

Printed in Great Britain by
Billing & Sons Limited, Guildford and London

Contents

To the memory of Timmy

General preface

This series is the first to approach the problem of language disability as a single field. It attempts to bring together areas of study which have traditionally been treated under separate headings, and to focus on the common problems of analysis, assessment and treatment which characterize them. Its scope therefore includes the specifically linguistic aspects of the work of such areas as speech therapy, remedial teaching, teaching of the deaf and educational psychology, as well as those aspects of mother-tongue and foreign-language teaching which pose similar problems. The research findings and practical techniques from each of these fields can inform the others, and we hope one of the main functions of this series will be to put people from one profession into contact with the analogous situations found in others.

It is therefore not a series about specific syndromes or educationally narrow problems. While the orientation of a volume is naturally towards a single main area, and reflects an author's background, it is editorial policy to ask authors to consider the implications of what they say for the fields with which they have not been primarily concerned. Nor is this a series about disability in general. The medical, social, educational and other factors which enter into a comprehensive evaluation of any problems will not be studied as ends in themselves, but only in so far as they bear directly on the understanding of the nature of the language behaviour involved. The aim is to provide a much needed emphasis on the description and analysis of language as such, and on the provision of specific techniques of therapy or remediation. In this way, we hope to bridge the gap between the theoretical discussion of 'causes' and the practical tasks of treatment—two sides of language disability which it is uncommon to see systematically related.

Despite restricting the area of disability to specifically linguistic matters—and in particular emphasizing problems of the production and comprehension of spoken language—it should be clear that the series' scope goes considerably beyond this. For the first books, we have selected topics which have been particularly neglected in recent years, and which seem most able to benefit from contemporary research in linguistics and its related disciplines, English studies, psychology, sociology and education. Each volume will put its subject matter in perspective, and will provide an introductory slant to its presentation. In this way, we hope to provide specialized studies which can be used as texts for components of teaching courses, as well as material that is directly applicable to the needs of professional workers. It is also hoped that this orientation will place the series within the reach of the interested layman—in particular, the parents or family of the linguistically disabled.

David Crystal
Jean Cooper

Preface

This book is essentially an attempt to introduce, describe and justify a grammatical assessment and remediation procedure that can be used with children or adults displaying some kind of language disability. In writing it, however, we have also found it necessary to incorporate two other kinds of information: for readers who have had little previous contact with studies of this general type, we have added background information about syntax, and about some of the main studies in syntactic abnormality that have been made in recent years; and for those well-versed in the literature on syntactic assessment, we have added points of comparison with our own procedure, and some degree of critique. The first two chapters, accordingly, present information and discussion which is at times introductory, at times technical. We have tried to maintain a reasonably smooth level of exposition by using footnotes for some of the more specialized comments and by a fairly frequent use of bibliographical references for elaboration of issues that we felt to be less central to our purposes. We have nonetheless been very aware of the difficulty of writing for two audiences at once, and we hope that the bringing together of these distinct expository modes will not prove unduly disconcerting. In our view, such problems are minor compared with the need to develop a critical and flexible attitude towards the use of syntactic procedures in remediation; and it is in the interests of developing this awareness that we have written our opening chapters in this way.

The book is the outcome of some ten years of work which progressed at various rates and intensities, and involved various stages of formulation and revision. It may therefore be helpful—especially to those teachers and therapists who have had some contact with this approach in courses and conferences in Great Britain—to be given a brief historical account of its development.

The Department of Linguistic Science was established at the University of Reading in 1965, and regular contact with the Audiology Unit of the Royal Berkshire Hospital began shortly afterwards. The period 1965–9 involved the first author observing and participating in speech therapy and audiology sessions at the RBH, out of which emerged various case studies and partial analyses. Simultaneously, the Department developed its teaching activities in this area, specifically in relation to the Diploma for the Teaching of Speech Therapy (Reading School of Education) and in its MA in Linguistics, on which speech therapists and mother-tongue teachers were beginning to be accepted. During this time also, in-service courses were taught by the first author to speech therapists and teachers in the Reading area on the relationship between linguistics and the remedial field, the general tone of which is summarized in Crystal 1972a. The demand for in-service lectures and courses became more insistent between 1969 and 1972, and culminated in a series of courses specifically on linguistics, langue acquisition and applied remedial work, held at Castle Priory College, Wallingford, Berkshire, throughout 1973 and 1974. For these courses, the decision was made to concentrate on syntax (for reasons explained in chapter 1), and a more intensive working-up of the syntactic approach followed. The third author had joined the Department as Lecturer in 1971, and the second author as a Canada MRC Research Fellow in 1973, thus allowing a more systematic application of the approach to a wider range of patients. A number of ex-Reading speech therapy students also began to use aspects of the approach in their work (e.g. Hutchison 1972). Adults were first systematically studied using the procedure in 1972, and between 1972 and 1974, the language assessment, remediation, and screening procedure (LARSP), as it came to be called, was introduced and discussed in relation to fields other than speech therapy—in particular, remedial teaching, the teaching of reading (Crystal 1973b, 1974a), special education, the teaching of the deaf (Crystal 1972b), and educational psychology. It is the widely found support for the approach, and interest in its application in these areas, which has led us to publish the present introduction, rather than wait a few more years for standardized data to become available. We are well aware of our limited experience. LARSP has been used systematically in detailed studies of some 30 children and 10 adults only, though a further 200 children and 50 adults have been studied in a more partial way. We have therefore been much reassured by our contact with clinicians, teachers, and others, that despite the acknowledged weaknesses, there seems to be a point in publishing an outline of the approach now.

We welcome discussion from readers about any aspect of our procedure, or its application in individual cases. Correspondence about the procedure as a whole should be addressed to the first author; further information about the case studies may be obtained from Dr Fletcher, who was primarily involved with chapter 7, and Dr Garman, for chapter 8. A tape-recording has been made illustrating the dialogues from these chapters, as well as the prosodic features involved. Information about this is obtainable from the authors. Further copies of the LARSP Profile Chart are also obtainable from the authors, University of Reading, White-knights, Reading RG6 2AA.

Our thanks are due to many people who have supported our interests over the past decade. In particular, without the willing cooperation and enthusiasm of Jennifer Schmit and Joan Telfer, the therapists involved in our main case studies, we would never have been able to progress so far in such a short time. The speech therapy staff at the Audiology Unit of the Royal Berkshire Hospital have displayed patience beyond measure in discussing their work with us, especially Ann Owlett, Ann Rundle and Pat Touche. Space unfortunately does not permit us to name all those who have helped us in various ways—especially by sending us material for analysis—from our local hospitals, the Reading and Berkshire Health Authorities, and schools and clinics up and down the country. But we should be at fault if we did not add a special work of thanks to Mr R. Hunt Williams and Dr Kevin Murphy, for introducing us to the work of the Audiology Unit, and allowing us to use their facilities, for the sympathy and assistance of Ray Johnson and Joyce Knowles of Castle Priory College, and to the participants on the courses they organized for counterbalancing our theories with their experience. We must also acknowledge our thanks to those colleagues in the Department of Linguistic Science who, while not being directly involved in this work, have nonetheless given generously of their time in criticizing earlier drafts of this book: Frank Palmer, Peter Matthews, Ron Brasington, David Wilkins, Peter Trudgill, Arthur Hughes, and Bill Hardcastle. Naturally, ours is the sole responsibility for the orientation and content of the final version.

Above all, to Mr J, and to the parents of Hugh, who gave permission for our intensive case studies to proceed, we are most grateful.

David Crystal
University of Reading
August 1974

1

The study of syntax

The neglect of syntax

Of all the points of contact between linguistics and those who work in the field of language abnormality, none has been more neglected until recently than the study of syntax. To the linguist, this is somewhat paradoxical. Work in general linguistics since the 1950s has clearly shown the indispensability of syntax in the analysis of human language. The two most influential books of the period reflect this concern in their titles: *Syntactic structures*, and *Aspects of the theory of syntax* (both by Noam Chomsky). And syntax has come to be seen as the network of organizational principles underlying linguistic expression, without which language would become an incoherent jumble of vocabulary and sound. It would accordingly be surprising if language disorders did not need to be related to syntax in some fundamental way; and it *is* surprising when one discovers how little attention has in fact been focused on this point.[1]

The indispensability of syntax is evident in the outline of most linguistic theories, which generally recognize three distinct aspects or *levels* in the study of language. These levels can be represented in the following way:

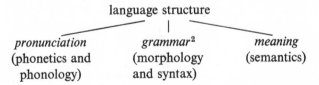

language structure

pronunciation	*grammar*[2]	*meaning*
(phonetics and	(morphology	(semantics)
phonology)	and syntax)	

[1] The neglect has been particularly apparent in Great Britain, where the work initiated by Menyuk, Lee and others in the 1960s seems to have had no influence on clinical training and practice. See further ch. 2, and for a convenient collection of relevant papers, Longhurst 1974.

[2] In this book the term *grammar* will be used to refer to all matters of structural organization exclusive of pronunciation and semantics. This is therefore a different use from that common in generative linguistics, where 'a grammar' of a language subsumes *all* these notions. Grammar for us comprises two subfields: morphology and syntax. The concept of the 'word' is at the centre of this distinction: morphology studies word structure (e.g. prefixes, suffixes, compounds, word-endings, or *accidence*); syntax studies the way in which sequences of words constitute larger patterns—phrases, clauses, and in particular, sentences and sentence-sequences. Our focus in this book is on syntax, but we shall be referring to morphology at various places, and whenever we do not wish to focus on the notion of syntax as such, the term *grammar* will be used. The common phrase, 'grammar and syntax', often used in the literature on disorders, for us has no meaning, therefore, and we recommend it should be avoided. Terminological caution is crucial: for example, Myklebust (1965) uses a 'syntax quotient' and finds it to be an unsatisfactory measure—but in fact he is dealing more with morphological errors under this heading.

There is currently a great deal of controversy about the relative importance of these levels, and how their interrelationships might best be seen. In particular, the relationship between syntax and semantics is undergoing much discussion (see, for example, McCawley 1968, Chomsky 1970). But despite this controversy, the usefulness of having the three above-named levels as focal points for theoretical and descriptive enquiry is generally recognized, and the central role of syntax, suggested by the model, is widely accepted. It is of course likely that, during the 1970s, arguments for the importance of semantics will be developed that will make the role of syntax seem less central, a more peripheral concern for the theoretical linguist. Such arguments tend to be of the following general kind: 'The communication of meaning is the primary purpose of language, and a linguistic theory ought to reflect this priority in its analytical models. Semantic analysis is at the heart of the matter; and the choice of syntactic expression in order to communicate our meanings is of secondary significance.' This approach may well be correct, but in practice it proves impossible to take account of it, at the present time. No semantic theory has been worked out sufficiently for descriptive studies of any general validity to have taken place; and the way in which semantic analyses are related to syntactic patterns is still highly controversial. As a result, while the study of language disorders can benefit from the occasional insights of the semantic approaches currently being developed, we are of the opinion that there is no chance of a theoretical or descriptive framework capable of application in a therapeutic or remedial context being evolved in the foreseeable future. We have consequently chosen to concentrate our efforts on the application of syntactic studies, where a great deal of theoretical and descriptive agreement is apparent. Our view of the centrality of syntax may then seem conservative to some from the point of view of linguistic theory; but from the point of view of clinical application, we claim it is realistic and necessary.

Our sense of paradox, then, results from the neglect of syntax at the expense of studies of pronunciation and vocabulary, especially the former. In speech therapy, the traditional focus of training in language has been in *phonetics* (the study of human soundmaking, in terms of articulation, acoustic transmission, and auditory reception) and, more recently, in *phonology* (the study of the sound systems of particular languages).[3] Training in syntax—or in other areas of linguistics, for that matter—was not given, and it was in fact only in 1974 that a syllabus in linguistics, paying introductory attention to syntax, was introduced by the College of Speech Therapists in Great Britain. In remedial education, the traditional focus has been on vocabulary enrichment, and semantic considerations generally; and the same applies to primary education as a whole, where studies of the reading process, for example, have concentrated on the two sides of the diagram above, ignoring the centre. The classical debate in the teaching of reading, for instance, is between the respective merits of 'phonic' and 'look-and-say' approaches, which is exclusively a matter of the left-hand side of the diagram—

[3] See O'Connor 1973 for a general account of these areas; for a discussion and application specifically to English, see Gimson 1970.

specifically, the way in which the phonological system can be related to its visual analogue:

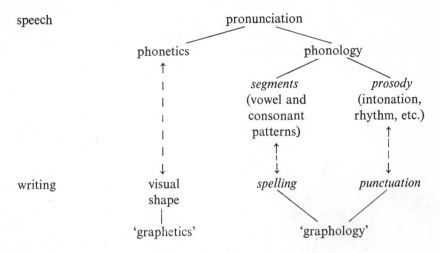

In a different connection, a great deal of time has been spent debating the question of vocabulary appropriateness, especially the selection of the proper vocabulary for children of specific socioeconomic backgrounds. But the whole field of grammar in the teaching of reading has, until very recently, been ignored.[4] We have also looked widely in the fields of mental subnormality and deaf education, to see whether the role of syntax in assessing the nature of a disability has been given proper emphasis and treatment; but again we have found little mention of it, and certainly only minimal attempts to think in terms of schemes of assessment and remediation based upon the findings of syntactic analysis. (The exceptions to this generalization will be reviewed in chapter 2.)

In all this, we are not saying that syntax has been *totally* ignored; but we do feel that its systematic importance has been quite underestimated, and that peripheral or superficial grammatical matters tend to be referred to at the expense of the more important underlying processes of sentence formation. The remainder of this chapter deals with four examples of what we consider to be a misplaced emphasis.

(i)   The focus on 'parts of speech'. The classical tradition of grammatical analysis handed down by the Greeks viewed language in terms of parts of speech, e.g. *noun, verb, conjunction*. In describing a language, the aim was to identify the part of speech a word belonged to, and then to present the various sequences permitted

---

[4] Schemes such as *Breakthrough to literacy* and *Link-up* (see MacKay, Thompson and Schaub 1970, Reid and Low 1973 respectively) have begun to take grammar into systematic account; but from the perspective of the grammatical information outlined later in this book, there is still a great deal yet to be considered. Compare, however, the aims of *Skylarks* (Bevington and Crystal 1975).

in the formation of sentence patterns. This emphasis permeated the whole of the traditional grammatical study of English, and it is reflected throughout the field of language development and language disorders. Most of the works on grammar referred to by McCarthy (1954), in her major review of child language studies, deal with the range and frequency of parts of speech in children (e.g. Davis 1938, Ellsworth 1951), there is a similar emphasis in work on adult aphasia (e.g. Jones, Goodman and Wepman 1963), and one often finds in contemporary therapy the (often implicit) principle of structuring a series of sessions in terms of parts of speech, e.g. working on prepositions one week, pronouns the next, and so on. The point that has to be made strongly is that this orientation, by itself, is inadequate as an account of language ability or disability. Grammar is far more than an ordered collection of parts of speech, and parts of speech constitute a very minor aspect of grammatical analysis and description when compared with the various processes of sentence construction. The reason is simple: the very definition of parts of speech depends on these processes. For example, if the question is asked 'What is a noun?', a generalized answer in grammatical terms[5] presupposes our knowledge of sentence-patterns, e.g. in English 'A noun is a word which may occur as the subject of a verb, as in *Dogs bark*', or 'A noun is a word which may occur "governed by" a preposition, as in *With luck . . .*', or 'A noun is a word which may be preceded by an article, as in *The boy . . .*'. We build up our definition of a noun by examining all the grammatical contexts in which words like *dog, boy, luck* are used; and the same procedure applies to all the other parts of speech. In other words, to focus on parts of speech without paying proper attention to the language's syntactic patterns is to put the cart before the horse. And if one is not aware of this, it is easy to confuse grammatical study by asking artificial questions and setting up irrelevant problems. For example, 'What part of speech is *round* really—preposition, adverb, noun . . . ?' The answer is: 'It depends on the context in which it occurs. If it occurs after an article, it is a noun; if it occurs before a noun, it is functioning as a preposition; and so on. There is no "basic" function to this word, such as is implied by the word "really".' Perhaps the most frustrated questions come from people who try to analyse the speech of very young children into 'parts', e.g. 'What part of speech is *allgone, ta, peep-bo, gimme . . .* ?' The enquirer is doomed to permanent frustration if he persists in putting the question in this form, for two reasons. Firstly, it is premature to ask such questions of young children's utterances, months before they have begun to develop word-uses capable of description in adult terms. Even with 'clearer' cases, like *want, shoe*, these words are at best only distant approximations to adult usage (see further, p. 64). And secondly, it is fallacious to assume that all words are capable of being assigned unambiguously to some traditional part of speech. Words like *hello, please, sorry* seem to defy classification in traditional terms, and need to be classified under fresh headings, if they are to be classified at all.

[5] Not in semantic terms, note. 'The noun is a name of a person, place, or thing' is a traditional answer, which tells us something about what a noun *means* (albeit rather vaguely), but gives us no information about what a noun *does* in the grammar of the language—where it goes in a sentence, whether it has case-endings etc.

For such reasons, attempts to count the number of parts of speech in a speech sample, or to ascertain the ratio of nouns to verbs, or nouns to adjectives, are going to produce at best partial, and at worst positively misleading results, if the analyst has been at all casual about his method of allocating words to the traditional labels (this tends to happen particularly frequently over the use of the label 'adverb'). Without careful attention to the bases of definition, one can never be sure that two analysts are in fact using a label in the same way—for example, whether 'proper names' (such as *London, John*) are being seen as nouns or as a separate part of speech—and comparing their linguistic descriptions (of two patients, for example) becomes at once an uncertain and ambiguous undertaking, unless one manages to find out exactly how they are using their descriptive labels. But as soon as they do give their formal criteria (which is not commonly done, in the traditional literature), this places the focus of attention fairly and squarely on the field of syntax.[6]

(ii) **The focus on length.** The length of a sentence or utterance is another measure often referred to in the literature on child development and disorders of language. It is a notion which, in various terminologies, has been in use for over half a century. MLR (mean length of response) is used by Nice (1925) and many others between 1930 and 1950 (see the review by McCarthy (1954)), the number of words per response being averaged over a given number of sentences, usually 50 in all. More recently, Roger Brown and his colleagues have developed a concept of MLU (mean length of utterance), based on the number of morphemes per utterance (see the specific instructions for calculation in Brown 1973, 54ff.). The trouble with measures of length is that they readily motivate the making of superficial judgements (though this is not a failing of Brown and his colleagues). It is true that sentence-length increases with age to some extent, but any single normative scale is very much an approximation, when one considers all the influencing factors. There is no neat linear development, especially between ages 3 and 5. Minifie *et al.* (1963) in fact argue that an index of length can be up to two years in error in either direction, as length is so readily affected by such variables as socioeconomic background, sex, IQ, and birth-order, as well as 'temporary' states such as health, emotion, the nature of the addressee, and so on. Cowan *et al.* (1967) showed how easy it is to establish bias in any length measure by varying the stimulus materials and the experimenter's role. Shriner (1967) finds MLR of little value over 5 because of increased response variability, and Brown (1973) does not use MLU after his stage V because by that time the child 'is able to make constructions of such great variety that *what* he happens to say and the MLU of a sample begin to depend more on the character of the interaction than on what the child knows,

[6] For a further discussion of word-classification, see Robins 1971, 216ff. and Crystal 1966. The need for criteria becomes more pressing as descriptive phrases become less specific and more impressionistic, e.g. a comment that a child's speech is getting 'less concrete' and 'more abstract' is intolerably vague without reference to formal criteria—and if concreteness reduces to (say) number of nouns and adjectives of a particular type, only reference to such criteria will permit consistency in making comparative assessments.

and so the index loses its value as an indicator of grammatical knowledge' (54).

Length by itself tells us very little. Two sentences may be exactly the same length, but internally be poles apart as regards their complexity. For example, most people would agree that the sentence *The man and the woman saw the cat and the dog* is less complex than *The man that the woman was speaking to saw the dog*, though both have the same number of words. The complexity would seem to be the important thing to try to pin down, and the notion of length therefore needs to be supplemented by a great deal more syntactic information. Apart from this, length is not as straightforward a thing to establish as may be thought. To begin with, there may be problems over identifying the unit which is being measured, e.g. if SENTENCES are being measured, does the analyst count all of the following as sentences? *Yes. In the morning* (said as response to the question *When will you arrive?*). *So much for that.* And how many sentences are there in utterances such as the following (taken from a 3-year-old's monologue while playing with his toys):

yes and it goes on here and it—and this one goes in the lorry and it goes up up up the hill and it goes up the hill—and it takes this all up the hill . . .

The difficulty is even more serious when it is UTTERANCES that are being measured, or RESPONSES, for it is far more difficult to define these notions than that of the sentence (and they rarely are defined in the papers we have read). This is one reason for caution, therefore. A further difficulty with length is that, even assuming that the units to be measured have been agreed, one still has to decide which units of measurement to use, and attempt to apply this measuring-rod consistently. There are many possible contenders for units of measurement—words, morphemes, intonation-units, syllables, stressed syllables, phonemes—and results will vary depending on which unit you choose. *The boys are running quickly* is longer than *The boy isn't running now* in terms of morphemes (*the - boy - s - are - run - ing - quick-ly; the - boy - is - n't - run - ing - now*), shorter in terms of the number of stressed syllables, and the same in terms of words. Moreover, each unit poses its own problems of applicability, e.g. in counting words, does one take contracted forms (*it's, isn't* etc.) as one word or two? Are idioms to be counted as separate words (e.g. is *spick and span* three words, even though the usage is fixed in this form)? There is also a whole history of problems in trying to make the notion of the morpheme work consistently in English. A morpheme is the smallest meaningful unit of grammatical form, and broadly corresponds to the notions of *root* and *affix* in traditional grammar. Most English words present little problem, when analysing them into morphemes: it is obvious that the word *blackbird* has two constituent morphemes, *black-* and *-bird*, and that *boys* has two morphemes *boy-* and *-s* (signalling the plural 'meaning'). But what does one do with *raspberry* (the constituent *-berry* is clearly identifiable, but what about *rasp-*?), *mice* (where the root *mouse* and the plural have somehow been fused), *sheep* (where the singular and plural forms are identical), and the many others? There are various possible answers to these questions, and in the 1940s the linguistics literature was full of debate about the alternatives.[7] Given such complexity, it is extremely difficult to

---

[7] See Joos 1957, or, for a recent review of the problems, Matthews 1974.

work consistently in establishing MLU in terms of morphemes, and results have to be viewed with caution.[8]

Length by itself is an inadequate indicator of grammatical ability, as Rees concludes (1971, 291): 'this procedure tends to obscure the nature of the child's grammatical skill as well as his efficiency in using language for expression and communication.' It has some methodological value, as a way of imposing a preliminary developmental ordering on samples of data, before carrying out a grammatical analysis, and this is the way in which it is used by Brown and his colleagues (see Brown 1973, Morehead and Ingram 1973, and other references there): 'two children matched for MLU are much more likely to have speech that is, on internal grounds, at the same level of constructional complexity than are two children of the same chronological age' (Brown 1973, 55). In this way, of course, it might be used as a screening test in a clinical context. Nor is there any reason why it should not be used along with a measure of complexity to produce a combined evaluation, e.g. Shriner's (1967) LCI (length-complexity index), which is a combination of MLR and various indices of structural complexity (after Templin 1957). But on its own, the data any length measure provides can be highly misleading. All there is in its favour is ease of applicability—a factor which is of no small value for the clinician or teacher pressed for time—and this has often led to its being used instead of sentence complexity (e.g. by Renfrew (n.d.)). But the question of optimum use of time makes sense only in the context of the long term, as we shall argue below (p. 24), and it is clear that in the long term, isolated measures of length can lead to faulty assessment and inappropriate choice of remediation techniques. To take two obvious problems, length will not differentiate between echolalic and novel speech; nor will it say anything about someone's ability to interact with his interlocutor in dialogue. Nor can length measures, by themselves, generate suggestions about specific therapeutic procedures. Getting the pupil or patient's (P)[9] sentences longer is a desirable aim, but the critical question is, How?

(iii)   Linguistic realism. It is essential to develop an accurate conception of the contemporary language, in any discussion of syntactic norms. Any procedure must allow direct comparison of the abnormal utterance with adult norms or the norms of children comparable in other respects, and T[9] must therefore be well aware of the nature of normal utterance, and use procedures capable of being applied with equal cogency to both normal and remedial speech situations. Most of the available syntactic assessment procedures seem to lack a normative dimension, in fact—something bemoaned by Longhurst and Schrandt in their review (1973, 248)—and we have ourselves often found Ts unsure of how a normal P would react when placed in a test situation of the kind T regularly uses. Perhaps the most

---

[8] The concept of MLR is reviewed by Shriner (1969), MLU by Crystal (1974b). Various measures are compared by Sharf (1972). Ingram (1972c) uses a combined length measure based on both words and morphemes.

[9] For convenience, we conflate the two main categories of remedial person under one heading. We shall do the same for teacher and therapist—T.

far-reaching misconception, in this respect, is for T to think of syntax purely or predominantly in terms of the written language, with speech being felt to have 'little' or 'no' or 'debased' grammar. This has been a particular hindrance in work with the hearing-impaired, where the problem of oral unintelligibility has led to a playing-down of the importance of syntax or judging its correctness solely in terms of written norms (see, for example, Heider and Heider 1940, Cooper 1967, and the review of the field by Pressnell 1973). But worries about allowing colloquial speech too major a role are widespread, in all areas of disability, though they sometimes appear in print in a rather indirect way, e.g. Muma 1971, 436, 'inasmuch as the data were obtained from oral samples, the contraction transformation is undoubtedly *spuriously* high' (our italics), which we read as a complaint about the frequency of such items as *don't, can't, isn't* etc.; or Lee and Canter (1971, 326), who say, in relation to *wanna, gonna, gotta* etc., that the child 'should not be penalized for this articulatory error.' These attitudes, whether consciously or unconsciously held, are not restricted to the field of language abnormality, of course. The entire Western grammatical tradition has only in this century begun to free itself from the rigid view that the written language enshrines the laws of correct grammatical expression, and that the spoken language should be made to conform to this (see Crystal 1971a for further discussion). But even these days there is still a reluctance to recognize the very considerable differences between the spoken and written forms of language, and syntactic remediation programmes, if they are not aware of these differences, inevitably suffer—sentence-structures become artificial, and misleading strategies are advocated. An example of artificiality in sentence structure may be found in the tendency to make sentences longer by symmetrical expansion of the elements of structure, e.g. Noun + Verb (NV) becomes NNV, then NNVV, then NNNVV, then NNNVVV, and so on, which rapidly produces absurd structures. Conn (1971) gets into difficulties over this, for instance. One of his sentences develops into *Jack and Jill are washing Jim and Jane*, to which a corresponding question stimulus is proposed: *Whom and whom are Jim and Jane washing?* An example of a mistake in strategy would be the attempt to eliminate the use of *and* as a means of linking sentences. This is something which is widely accepted as an appropriate stylistic correction in the written language of children, and on the basis of this it has been said to be an appropriate correction for speech too, and an improper feature to reinforce in therapy. Lee and Canter, for example, say (1971, 329): 'Since there is no grammatical constraint on the endless use of conjunctions, special rules had to be created to avoid deceptively long, high-scoring sentences.' Only one *and* per sentence at clause level is accordingly allowed, and 'This treatment may be given to any other *overused* conjunctions' (our italics). But at the appropriate linguistic age (around 3 years, see p. 76, reinforcement of *and*, and other sentence-linking features of this kind, we find to be one of the most important strategies to advocate (see also Hutchison 1972).

It is important, too, to be familiar with the extent of 'normal nonfluency' in colloquial speech (see Crystal and Davy 1969, 104), and the range of variations in colloquial usage which affect the definition of syntactic rules. Deciding on the acceptability of a sentence is not a hard-and-fast matter (see Quirk and Svartvik

1966). In this respect, therefore, we find the 'all-or-none' scoring technique—as used by Lee and Canter (1971), for example—too inflexible, as it does not allow for the varying degrees of grammatical completeness which we find to be a regular feature of the speech of children at certain ages. Lee and Canter say, for instance: 'A structure is not given a score unless all the required syntactic and morphological rules have been observed. No intermediate steps are credited' (317). For example, pronouns need *all* of the features of person, number, gender and case before a score is allowed—*mine car*, for instance, would score 0. They do allow some colloquial reductions, but only if they conform to the structural patterns assumed as a general model; for example, usages like *I can* 'qualify as sentences since they contain both subject and predicate. While the verbs are incomplete, they are not exactly incorrect in a conversational, spontaneous speech sample' (325). But the majority of the elliptical patterns of spontaneous speech are not allowed, and there is accordingly a marked bias against colloquial speech in the scoring.[10] Intonational questions—to take a further example—are 'scored as incorrect questions'. We therefore doubt the conclusion that their technique 'allows a clinician to estimate the child's ability to formulate and produce grammatically "loaded" sentences *in the kind of conversational setting which he encounters daily* with his parents, his teachers, and his peers' (337, our italics).[11]

In short, any syntactic procedure must be firmly grounded in the facts of both written and spoken usage, and of the various styles (formal, informal etc.) and dialects subsumed under these two headings. But above all, the approach must pay proper regard to the facts of colloquial speech—the most frequently used variety of adult language, and the one children hear most consistently during their linguistically formative years. This principle is worth emphasizing as it is frequently transgressed. Bizarre syntax is common in both test materials and reading schemes. In the Northwestern, for example, there is the distinction between *The man brings*

[10] A reluctance to accept elliptical patterns is quite common in traditional grammar, and turns up frequently in applied linguistic studies. Another example is Sharf (1972, 66), who excludes from his samples any specific replies to questions: 'fill-in answers' 'were excluded on the basis that they were not expressive of spontaneous grammatical construction.' But knowledge of what to omit is an important aspect of linguistic creativity (see further below).

[11] On more general grounds, we see important limitations in approaches (such as in the Northwestern Syntax Screening Test) which permit the occurrence of error always to outrank the presence of positive structural ability. The instructions to that test say: 'Any change of the examiner's spoken sentence which affects the test item is considered a failure, even though the child's response is grammatically and semantically correct' (Lee 1969, 5), and 'Any response which contains a grammatical error, even though it is not the test item, is considered a failure on the grounds that the test item, though correct, may have introduced enough complexity to cause other structures to be dropped' (6). But how can this view conceivably be validated? On what linguistic grounds should the correct or incorrect use of -*s* in the verb, for example, affect the use of a determiner in the subject noun-phrase? Lee 1969 is only a screening test, not a general assessment, but a screening test which does not bring out areas of strength as well as areas of weakness is likely to produce a distorted picture. Contrast Dever (1972a, 1973), where phrase level error 'cannot affect clause level classification' (Dever and Bauman 1971, 25) and vice versa. (We would not go as far as Dever and Bauman, however, in saying that 'when a child gives an *incorrect* response we know nothing' (6).)

the boy the girl and *The man brings the girl the boy*. There too most of the sentences make use of the present tense (e.g. *The boy jumps*), which is a relatively uncommon usage. Overuse of this tense-form is a dominant feature of reading schemes also. Some examples of odd syntax from such schemes: *What have you in the shop?* (an archaic usage, where these days we would say *What have you got* etc.), *One kitten runs to the basket* (strange use of an emphatic determiner in an unemphatic context, and a 'sports commentary' present tense again), and *One little, two little, three little kittens*. Some of these sentences would be acceptable with appropriate intonation, of course (e.g. nursery-rhyme intonation for the last example), but we have not noticed such intonations to be a regular feature of T's or P's performance in the teaching situation.

(iv) Selective commentary. We suggested above that reference to syntax has not been adequately systematic in the literature on disorders. What we note now is a readiness to *list* information about syntactic features, without relating this inventory to some general framework. Almost any case study or longitudinal comparison of Ps will demonstrate this. The following extract is taken at random from a recent Journal (it is in fact a study which is well above average in its syntactic awareness, and where the author makes it quite clear that there is a great deal left unsaid):

> The same patient, D.Ed, retained his severe agrammatism, to use the traditional term, long after his active lexicon had multiplied many times. His early difficulty in using verbal forms—or anything other than substantives—has been mentioned. This was fairly resistant to efforts on the therapist's part to prevent the development of telegraphic speech: language habilitation centered on helping the patient to produce various simple syntactic patterns such as imperative forms . . . descriptions like 'It's heavy' . . . in answer to questions of the type of 'What's the hammer like?' . . . He could be helped to retrieve or acquire adjectives fairly soon after the nouns, but there long remained difficulty in combining the two. . . . The inclusion of a preposition to effect a linguistic relationship was difficult. . . . He frequently omitted articles, and, which interfered more with communication, the auxiliary 'is', or 'was' in verbs. . . . (Hatfield 1972, 76)

This quotation does not do justice to the sensitivity, balance and illustrative detail of this paper, but it does show the limitations of its method. This kind of selective commentary is easy enough to do, if one has had any kind of exposure to grammatical tradition, and it can spark off ideas. But it is of dubious value as an instructional or remedial method, because it fails to relate its observations to some general perspective, without which any linguistic profile is inevitably arbitrary. Comparison with other Ps is difficult because of the idiosyncratic selection and ordering of the data (the movement from verbs to adjectives to prepositions to articles etc. in the above quotation is unlikely to have been motivated by any theoretical considerations). Assessment on the basis of such an inventory is unreliable, because there is no guarantee that one has spotted the most important syntactic processes, and there would be an inevitable tendency to pick on those features of syntax which are the most readily describable, e.g. pronouns, omission of grammatical words, such as *the, of*. Nor is remediation assisted, as here one needs to be systematically aware of what P has *not* got in syntax, before choosing an area on which to work; but given an inventory of what is present in a sample of P's speech—even if this is an exhaustive account of the sample—it is left up to the analyst (or reader interested in using the results) to work out for himself what is not, and this is an extremely difficult and irritating task. The same criticism applies to syntactic assessment procedures which use only a small selection of features of syntax: the question has to be asked, Why these and not others? Has the selection been made on a principled basis, or is it impressionistic? For example, when Reynell (1969) isolates pronouns, prepositions, conjunctions, and questions (other than intonational) as four categories to be scored (item 11 on the Expressive Developmental Language Scale), one wants to know on what grounds this particular selection of features was made (see further, p. 18). Or again, is the concentration on morphological data and 'function words' in the well-known tests, and the exclusion of more general tests of syntactic ability, a decision of principle on the part of the authors? (See, for example, the Grammatic Closure Sub-Test of the Illinois Test of Psycholinguistic Abilities (Kirk and Kirk 1971, Kirk, McCarthy and Kirk 1968), or Lerea 1958 with reference to the Michigan Picture Language Inventory.)

Such questions abound when one considers the literature on language disorders. They can be answered only by developing what, for lack of a better term, we can call a proper degree of 'syntax-awareness', and this means relating any commentary to some descriptive framework which deals comprehensively and systematically with the syntactic features of the language—in other words, a 'grammar'. Only then will generalizations about someone's competence or incompetence in syntax be able to be assessed, compared, and implemented. We therefore isolate as two central goals for any work on remedial syntax that it be (*a*) in principle, comprehensive, and (*b*) systematic. And of the two, it is the need to be aware of system which is crucial. One *could* produce a comprehensive inventory of the syntactic features of a language; but an inventory provides no explanation, or sense of underlying pattern. To have a list of features, in which item 13 was the definite article, and item 97 the indefinite article would be of little value. At some point in any grammar of English, these two items have to be brought together, and their complementarity of function investigated. And so it is for all aspects of grammar. Grammar is not a random collection of features, nor is it learned in this way (see chapter 4). It is a highly complex system of structures and meanings, and doing a syntactic analysis means establishing how the various patterns in speech can be located within this overall system. It is the task of the grammarian to define all the variables which operate within this system, and to suggest an optimum route by means of which all aspects of the grammar can be displayed and interrelated. There are many possible methods of grammatical analysis available (our own being presented in chapter 3). But it should be clear that without some attempt at a comprehensive and systematic procedure, the dangers of an uncontrolled impressionism come to the fore, and the possibility of carrying out objective and consistent comparative work considerably recedes.

It is at this point that the role of the linguist becomes clear. Establishing a grammatical analysis that is unambiguous and comprehensive is a specialist, time-

and space-consuming task, and the value of much recent published work on syntactic disorders is diminished by authors not being fully aware of this. It is simply not possible to do a clinical investigation of a group of Ps *and* present a grammatical framework in the course of a few pages, but this is what is regularly attempted in the journals. The likelihood is that the grammatical model will be explained in an approximate or oversimplified way, with only a small proportion of structures and descriptive labels being selected and properly illustrated, and apparently arbitrary distinctions being made, in the absence of any discussion of criteria. For example, Engler *et al.* (1973), in an analysis that is far more detailed and discriminating than most (and which, incidentally, seems to parallel ours in many ways, cf. below), presents a skeleton analysis of syntactic structures that is of very limited use. There is one main reason for this. It has no mention of criteria,[12] and thus the reader is left unclear as to the grounds on which a distinction has been made, and how many other cases of a similar kind there might be. At one point, for example, they say that in Subject–Verb–Object constructions, the intensive verb is subclassified into three types: 'complement taking' (e.g. *look, seem*), 'senses intransitive' (e.g. *taste*), and 'middle' (e.g. *weigh*). The reader who wishes to use their system of analysis, however, is left quite in the dark. How many other verbs like *weigh* are there? How do you decide whether a verb is 'middle' or not? Nor are Engler *et al.* atypical in their inexplicitness. Longhurst and Schrandt, for example, have a paper comparing the merits of four assessment procedures in respect of their ease of applicability (how much technical linguistics was needed, and whether the instructions were clear), inter-scorer reliability, ability to discriminate language differences between children, and ability to describe these differences. They conclude (1973, 248): 'None of the four linguistic procedures investigated [*sc* Lee and Canter 1971, Engler *et al.* 1973, Dever and Bauman 1971, Lee 1966] proved to be completely explicit and sufficient for analysing the speech of children', and the same applies to other papers that we have read in this area (e.g. Braun and Klassen 1971). Approaches which explicitly refer to some grammatical theory are strongest in these respects, e.g. those which base themselves on a particular model of transformational grammar (such as Menyuk (1963) in her use of Chomsky (1957a); or Morehead and Ingram's (1973) use and modification of Rosenbaum's (1967) adaptation of Chomsky (1965); or Dever (1972a, 1973), who uses tagmemic analysis). But even these approaches are extremely selective in their illustration of grammatical features and processes,[13] so that it proves difficult or impossible for T to 'follow the model' and use it for himself. T is continually being left to make his own decisions about questions of analysis—

[12] Apart from a footnote stating that there is a problem over deciding whether a construction is a passive or an adjectival complement. But they do not say what the problem is, or how it is to be resolved.

[13] Morehead and Ingram (1973) find that their grammars accounted for all but 8–10 per cent of the sampled utterances—but their sample was relatively small, as is suggested by some of their results for the normal sample, e.g. (in their terms) *all, vocative* and *stative verb particle-shift* (e.g. *up ball*) transformations are never used after their stage I, prepositions after stage II, *Verb qualifiers* (e.g. *I just go*) after stage I until stage V; *object noun retention* (e.g. *hit it ball*) is used only in stage II, and *inchoative* (e.g. *it got red*) only in stage III.

whether an item should be analysed as X or Y—particularly as regards the more restricted grammatical patterns. And for those approaches which do *not* relate to any accepted linguistic theory, the problem for the reader is far worse.

It should be noted that this criticism is a very specific one. It is not a criticism of the various methods when used by their respective authors; but it *is* certainly a criticism of the usefulness of the approaches, for unless such work is sufficiently explicit to be generally usable, one wonders why it was published in the first place. There is, however, only one way to avoid this criticism (apart from turning one's papers into a book—as in fact has been done by Dever (1972a) and Lee (1974)). It is impossible to present the entirety of a syntactic system in any meaningful way in a few pages *unless one can relate one's outline to some established grammatical canon.* In this way the clinician is relieved of the responsibility to have to explain all his descriptive apparatus, or deal with problem areas, as these will be given full discussion at the appropriate point in the grammatical tradition on which he is relying. The problem for the clinician, of course, is then to make a good choice of a grammar, and we shall have more to say on this in chapter 2. But this aside, we have been surprised to find that workers in the field of syntactic disorders have rarely tried to relate their work to conventional descriptive grammars of English. The problem of explanatory clarity thus remains.

A related criticism would fall under the heading of *representativeness*. It may be impossible for a syntactic procedure intended for remediation use to incorporate information of a maximally detailed kind, but at least all the main areas of grammar should be given some recognition, and a balance kept regarding the depth of detail of the description presented. Procedures which go into great detail about, say, morphology, but tell us little or nothing about phrase structure would be clear cases for criticism. One of the criticisms we have of Lee's method of Developmental Sentence Scoring (1966, 1969)[14] falls under this heading—though here the strength of the approach is in fact in its information about phrase structure. She selects eight syntactic features to score: (i) indefinite pronouns or noun modifiers (e.g. *this, some, each*), (ii) personal pronouns (e.g. *me, your, myself, who*), (iii) main verbs (e.g. *see, is, may, have*), (iv) secondary verbs (e.g. *going to*, I like *swimming,* I want *to go*), (v) negatives (e.g. *not, isn't*), (vi) conjunctions (e.g. *and, because, than*), (vii) interrogative reversals (e.g. *is it, could he . . .*), (viii) *wh*-questions (e.g. *what, how . . .*). Now while we accept that, for her purposes, to score every feature in the grammar would be 'clinically impractical' (1971, 319), we nonetheless find her particular selection to be unrepresentative of the syntactic system as a whole, and think that she has been unnecessarily dismissive of other areas of syntax which we hold to be of critical significance in assessing the character of a language disorder—in particular, the order of elements in clause and noun-phrase structure. Lee lists a number of the features not scored separately: 'the use of articles, plurals, possessive markers, prepositional phrases, adverbs, word order, word selection . . .' and says, 'To account, at least in part, for these unscored items, an additional

[14] See also Lee and Canter 1971. The approach is reviewed by Bloom (1967), Longhurst and Schrandt (1973), and Tyack (1972b). See pp. 196–7 below for some comments on Lee's most recent publication (1974).

sentence point is added to the total sentence score if the entire sentence is correct in all respects' (Lee and Canter 1971, 320). We find such an allocation to a child who can command all such features miserly in the extreme![15] Putting this another way, we find it unsatisfactory that sentences such as *Boy eat* or *Boy eat cookie* would each score 0 using her procedure—in our view a complete reversal of linguistic priorities. (It may be contrasted, for example, with the separate attention given to the various 'processes of arrangement' in Engler *et al.* 1973.) Another example of selectivity is Reynell's Expressive Language Scale. This is largely concerned with distinctions in length and quantity, but a few structural features are incorporated. These however are categorized too generally (e.g.'word combinations', 'correct use of words in sentences', 'use of subordinate clauses'), and in the one case where specific structures are cited, we cannot understand the basis of selection, from the point of view of developmental progress (see chapter 4). One point is scored for correct use of any three of pronouns, prepositions, conjunctions, and questions other than intonational. But prepositions emerge as early as Stage II in the classification in chapter 4; pronouns develop over a period from Stage III to Stage VI; formal questions are concentrated in Stages II–IV, and conjunctions are the dominant constructional process at Stage V. To score 1 for any 3 seems a strange juxtaposition of values.

Lastly, concerning the problems of selective commentary, it is important to ensure that any information obtained through the use of the syntactic procedure is retained in the final presentation of the results, so that a balanced and wide-ranging picture may be had of P's ability in the syntactic system as a whole. Bearing in mind the number of major variables which have to be taken into account, we therefore take the view that any attempt to work out a single syntactic 'score' is going to be of negligible diagnostic or therapeutic value, in respect of the above desiderata. Syntax scores have often been tried, e.g. Lee 1966, Brannon and Murry 1966, Reynell 1969; but we have found them unilluminating, and at times counter-intuitive. Sometimes, even, we have the impression that the internal logic of the scoring system takes over the linguistic analysis, and forces linguistically questionable rules or classifications, e.g. Lee and Canter (1971, 325) find themselves in danger of overscoring words like 'it was *broken*', so they assume that these are learned as adjectives: 'a rule was made that if the past participle verb form could be used as an adjective in a noun phrase, the sentence would be scored as copula + adjective, not as a passive'.[16] Scores will become more useful only when

[15] For these reasons we are not surprised to see Sharf's conclusion (1972). He compared four measures of language development (MLR, NDW (number of different words), LCI (length-complexity index) and DSS (developmental sentence scoring) and finds a close correlation between the first two and the last two. He concludes that for relating language growth to chronological age, 'it appears that quantification of structural analysis of language provides no more sensitive measure than quantification of verbal output' (73)—though he accepts that the former are of no remedial use. But this may be no more than a comment on the limitations of the structural analyses cited.

[16] Cf. above p. 12 for the similar difficulty over coordination. In a different, but related connection, we note that the listing of transformations is sometimes carried out regardless of their diagnostic relevance: e.g. Morehead and Ingram give a number of categories which seem to have little or no role in their subsequent analysis, some of which are listed in fn. 13 above.

the influence of extralinguistic factors (such as class and sex) on syntax comes to be better understood, and the concept of a 'matched' sample made more plausible. For the time being, therefore, we prefer to avoid the notion of a score, and think instead in terms of a syntactic profile (see below), in which a wide range of syntactic variables are simultaneously presented, and a qualitative assessment made of the areas of strength and weakness. The integrated set of values present in the profile could of course be given a statistical analysis, and this will be an important feature of any standardization of this procedure; but for routine remedial work, we have found this to be unnecessary.

2

Some critical factors in devising a syntactic remediation procedure

A consideration of the weaknesses in the traditional study of syntax in language disorders naturally suggests the areas which any positive contribution to this field would need to concentrate on. But before going into the specific characteristics of a syntactic procedure, it is important to consider in general terms what the purpose of the exercise is. What exactly do we expect such a procedure to be able to do? We therefore begin with a statement of aims.

Aims

Our aim is to develop a procedure for analysing the syntactic character of language disorders, capable of being used routinely by anyone involved with the diagnosis, assessment and remediation of language disability. Such a procedure would fulfil a variety of functions, of which we see the following as being the most central.

(*i*)   It must be capable of providing a framework for use as a screening procedure, i.e. as a technique for determining whether or not there is a case for more systematic linguistic examination.

(*ii*)   It must be able to provide a comprehensive description of P's syntactic output at any stage during the processes of assessment and diagnosis.

(*iii*)   It must be able to provide a principled therapeutic methodology.

Points (*ii*) and (*iii*) are fundamental, and need further discussion.

Concerning (*ii*), implicit at any stage is a comparison between the syntactic patterns P *has* and those he *should* have. T must work within an integrated developmental perspective—by which we mean, in practical terms, that he must know where he is at any given point in treatment. There are two sides to this, though: (*a*) knowing what structures *have* been acquired (and with what degree of mastery), and (*b*) knowing what structures have *not* been acquired but which would be appropriate for the stage of development that P seems to be at. This second point is perhaps the most underestimated in clinical language programmes, and unless one is aware of its implications, problems rapidly accumulate without being noticed. T takes a structure, and after training, P makes progress in its use. As a result, T develops the use of this structure, building on it and extending it in various ways, and there is further progress. But caution is necessary. This is only one structure among a number that P may need to develop. By concentrating on one to the exclusion of the others, T runs the risk of developing an unbalanced linguistic skill, and of overestimating P's syntactic ability. T has to make himself aware of the entire range of structures that ought to be developing at any given stage, so that he knows clearly what he has *not* taught as well as what he has. It is sometimes difficult for T to *stop* working with a structure that has been successfully introduced to P, and to turn to something else, but such decisions are crucial if a balanced syntactic skill is to emerge.[1]

There are other aspects of the need for T to have available a comprehensive descriptive picture of P, at any given stage. One is to be able to evaluate the unexpected structure, when it arises. A typical situation, we find, is for T to be concentrating on eliciting a particular structure, and P comes out with a different structure. The problem for T is to decide what to do with this: should it be ignored, reinforced, modified? Such a decision can only be made, however, if T is able to see how this structure relates to the others that have been used or taught, and those yet to be introduced. Any syntactic procedure, to be of use, must allow this kind of ready cross-checking. A second aspect of this situation is to enable a systematic revision or recapitulation to take place between remedial sessions, or whenever a period of time elapses between assessments. A checklist of syntactic patterns, properly organized, we find is especially important when we are faced with apparent regression in behaviour. With dysphasic adults, for example, variations in clinical and mental condition are so frequent that it is essential to be able to plot with some precision the various rises and falls in syntactic ability, otherwise therapy rapidly becomes random and impressionistic.

Concerning point (*iii*), the provision of a principled therapeutic methodology, we see this as the corollary of our second aim. A grammatical analysis of a disordered individual, by itself, is of restricted value.[2] What T needs to know is how to proceed, once the character of the syntactic disability has been determined. Any system of syntactic analysis which is to be of remedial value must be organized in such a way that some grading of structures is apparent. When should a particular structure be introduced into a remediation programme? When should it be phased out? What alternative structures can be used, if P fails to respond to one's first choice? What is the optimum route through the syntactic system (or, if there is no optimum route, what are the routes most likely to be successful)? Such questions are central, and in providing answers, it is important that the principles underlying any procedure should be made quite explicit. Unless T can answer the question 'Why?' in all of this, there is a real danger of remediation degenerating into a mechanical routine.

Aims (*ii*) and (*iii*) between them constitute a demand for an integrated perspective

---

[1] In one case, just such an imbalance had been created due to therapy having concentrated on the use of specific parts of speech and phrases. When Peter (aged 4½) was first referred to us, he had a good range of noun-phrases, verb phrases, prepositional phrases etc., but next to no awareness of the main elements of sentence structure, so that his phrases came out with little relationship to each other, and a resulting ambiguity and unintelligibility. Subsequent therapy had to redress the balance, by concentrating on sentence structure.

[2] It is this point which we find constitutes the main difficulty with many of the syntactic analyses intended for remediation, e.g. Myerson and Goodglass 1972. To write 'a grammar' of a patient is only the first stage.

in studying syntactic disability, without which we do not feel T can proceed with confidence. It is this, the establishment of confidence in remedial decision-making, with which we are ultimately concerned, and as one prerequisite for confidence is knowing the limitations, as well as the strengths, of a procedure, we should make it clear from the beginning of this book that there are certain clinical decisions involving linguistic reasoning to which we find it impossible to make any contribution, in the present state of knowledge. In particular, we are not ready to make any systematic contribution to questions of diagnosis, and this is why we do not cite diagnosis as one of our primary aims. It is unfortunately the case that insufficient Ps have been analysed in terms of syntax to enable any general categorization to be made, other than in the broadest terms (see chapter 6). We share in the widely voiced criticism of some of the general labels that have been used to characterize linguistic disturbance (e.g. 'agrammatism') that they are too inspecific to be of practical use, or leave unclear whether the deficit is to be identified primarily in linguistic or nonlinguistic (e.g. cognitive) terms; and we do not propose to add to this confusion by constructing a further set of vaguely defined and empirically unsupported categories for syntax. Once the appropriate amount of empirical spadework has been carried out, and a normative framework established, we hope to hazard a classification of syntactic disturbances which may be of diagnostic value. But for the present, our entire orientation is towards the individual, and away from the group. We wish to establish progress in P's syntax, and to control it. Only after this has been done in many cases can we compare individual strategies and responses, and suggest typologies. In this we find ourselves at one with Rosenthal *et al.* (1972) who, after evaluating seven major diagnostic categories, and finding them all to be heterogeneous and ambiguous, also conclude: 'assessment ought to be aimed at determining individual treatment needs, and not toward assignment of the child to a specific diagnostic category' (135). The same applies to work with adults.

Desiderata

We have so far talked in very general terms about syntax and its application in remedial work, but we have also at times referred to specific procedures, by way of illustration. We now propose to look more thoroughly at what we feel to be the basic factors that need to be borne in mind in constructing any syntactic remedial procedure. It is clear that developing such a procedure is going to be no easy matter, when one looks at the range of considerations, theoretical and practical, linguistic and nonlinguistic, that affect the issue, and we have not been surprised to find that none of the available approaches satisfactorily meet the criteria that we consider central. We have all of us learned a great deal from the work cited in this chapter and in chapter 1, most of which was developed in the United States in the mid-1960s; but we have been unable or unwilling to use this in our own work, and we must explain why, as a preliminary to outlining our own approach later in the book. We propose to do this by isolating certain general principles, to which we think any syntactic procedure should conform.

(i) General applicability. The model developed must be capable of being applied (*a*) to both normal and disordered individuals, (*b*) to problems both of assessment and remediation, (*c*) to both adult and child Ps, in all the domains of remedial work,[3] and (*d*) to the analysis of both comprehension and production. We shall comment briefly on each of these points.

(*a*) The model, as we have already suggested, must be comprehensive, to allow for routine comparison with normal development, at whatever stage. But there is a second reason why any model cannot set its sights lower than a full grammar of the adult language, and that is because very often the focus of T's attention must be on *his own* syntax. This is particularly so when the disorder is severe, when little expressive language is being produced, or where there is a comprehension problem. In such cases the syntactic procedure swings round to operate on T's use of language. And generally in remediation, awareness of one's own syntactic habits is an essential feature of any evaluation of progress.

(*b*) One of the main points to emerge from the discussion so far is the need to maintain a proper balance in any clinical procedure between assessment and remediation. This means, in linguistic terms, that the procedure has to be evaluated according to the attention it pays to its system of syntactic description and to its system of grading structures; and we shall discuss both these points in detail below. The main difficulty we have had with the approaches we have studied, however, is that on the whole they do not maintain this balance: they are either systems of assessment and diagnosis, with implications for remediation, or they are remedial programmes, lacking perspective in assessment. The most successful attempts to preserve a balance, in our opinion, are those by Lee, Dever, Ingram, and their associates, and we shall frequently be referring to their work, by way of comparison with our own. The general point we would make is that it is not possible to integrate the elements of assessment and remediation without relating one's procedure to some specific grammatical approach and some specific scale of development.

(*c*) The procedure should not insist on a rigid distinction between adult and child syntax. The essential continuity of development from child to adult argues against it, and any such division would give rise to all kinds of practical difficulties, e.g. should one use the adult or the child procedure in analysing the language of adolescents in special education? At a more detailed level of argument, we have noted some approaches where the procedures are inapplicable (without modification) to certain clinical populations. Dever (1972a), for example, takes for granted the use of well-defined intonational units at the beginning of his syntactic remediation procedure TALK (Teaching the American Language to Kids), and his system thus cannot be readily used for children whose initial difficulties are largely

---

[3] Here we are referring to the traditional interdisciplinary barriers, which have been very marked in remedial work. The subject of language disability is of interest to many groups— clinicians, mother-tongue teachers, and foreign-language teachers, in particular. The remarkable thing is that each of these has its own journals, conferences etc., which members of the other groups rarely encounter. The points of contact between these fields need to be explored, materials shared, and duplication of work avoided.

prosodic (as with certain ESN and 'non-communicating' children, for example) and for many adult dysphasics.

(*d*) The procedure should be capable of being used in the study of disorders of both production and comprehension. Of the two, we feel that the main gap is in the field of production, and it is there that we see a syntactic procedure as being most beneficial. We have accordingly biased our presentation in that direction. But it should be clear that in principle the procedure could be used as a means of structuring and grading sentence patterns for comprehension work, or in trying to establish what range of patterns promoted comprehension difficulties, and we have noted significant similarities between our own approach and some of the work on comprehension, e.g. Mittler *et al.* 1974. (We do not however assume that production and comprehension develop in parallel: see below, and also Clark *et al.* 1974.)

(ii) Clinical realism. If it is to be convincing, a syntactic procedure must be able to identify the character of a disorder fairly directly and systematically, and should not regularly conflict with the intuition of the experienced T concerning the degree of delay or severity that may be present. It must also be able to cope with the description of the range of abnormal linguistic patterns used by P. At a more everyday level, it must be capable of being learned by T with a minimum of linguistic training, and capable of being used bearing in mind the pressures of the clinical or teaching situations.

This last point needs to be amplified, as there is inevitably a tension between accuracy and comprehensiveness on the one hand and speed and simplicity of use on the other. This applies to a syntactic analytic procedure as much as to any other, and it is up to T to judge how best to arrive at the optimum balance between time spent on matters of analysis and interpretation, and time spent in actual therapy or teaching. The hard fact of the matter is that if one wants to achieve a complete and accurate understanding of a syntactic disability, there is no alternative but to spend analytic time on it—perhaps 3 or 4 hours, in order to obtain a reasonably full analysis of a half-hour sample (see chapter 5). Many Ts obviously find such an outlay of time impossible, as a routine enterprise, and, unfortunately, opt for techniques which may be less helpful but are more practicable. The sad story of the *Bus Story* is a case in point. Renfrew's original method was found to be unreliable, and so: 'Eventually it was abandoned in favour of a scheme based on transformational grammar and devised by a psycholinguist. This method, though in many ways more satisfactory, proved time consuming and required considerable practice to achieve consistent results. The busy clinician, for whom the scale was being devised, rejected it on account of its complexity' (Renfrew n.d., 14–15), and went instead for a measure of sentence length. Not all methods of syntactic analysis pose such problems of complexity, consistency and time as transformational ones, of course, but the principle at stake here is a general one: simple analyses of complex phenomena only postpone problems; they do not solve them, and they may obscure them. However, with the best will in the world, it is often simply impossible for T to carry out even a reduced analysis of even his most interesting and problematic cases, because of pressure of time. In such situations, the only real solution is long-term—an improvement in the T:P ratio, and a more realistic job-analysis which pays due attention to the complexity of this kind of assessment and allows appropriate time to be given to it.[4] (In the short-term, it is possible for T to be helped if he can enlist the services of a tame linguist to do the analyses for him.)[5] In relation to the question of time, though, we would make two points:

(a) T should bear in mind that while any syntactic technique seems complex and cumbersome on first acquaintance, familiarity and practice promote acceptability. Also, it will not prove necessary to practise any technique with the utmost attention to detail on all occasions. Anyone who uses the procedure described in this book (or any other) more than three or four times will find that he has developed an intuition about the *kind* of syntactic pattern likely to be important, and will be able to make rapid and reasonably reliable judgements about syntactic abnormality without having to work systematically through the entire procedure. But having said this, there is no gainsaying that initial mastery of the technique will take time: there is no quick and easy way to learn syntactic analysis.

(b) But the problem of time must be put in perspective, and assessed over the long-term, in relation to the total anticipated contact time between T and P. The argument here is that time used in analysis and interpretation in the *early* stages of remediation is likely to save time later on, and obtain more definite progress in the meantime. We have seen the situation obtain repeatedly, particularly in adult dysphasia clinics, where many hours are spent in maintaining a good degree of personal contact between therapist and patient, but with little overall linguistic progress being achieved, due to no time having been put aside for the systematic analysis of each patient's problems. We hope there will develop an increased awareness of the essential role of analysis and interpretation sessions in providing a remediation service, as we see this, in the long run, as being one of the main ways in which clinical time can be saved.

(iii) Gradability. The structural features of the model must be presented in terms of some explicit principle of developmental progress, if a systematic remediation procedure is to emerge. The question is, Which? Our answer is on broadly similar lines to that of Norma Rees (1971), in a paper on the bases for decision in language training. She reviews six possible methods, and we follow her classification.

(a) The first—and in many ways the most obvious—is to organize structures in terms of some independent measure of complexity, and a number of attempts have been made to do this, mainly working within the framework of generative

[4] There is a natural but regrettable tendency to underestimate the time needed to do clinically usable linguistic analyses. The Quirk Report (London, Department of Education and Science, 1972), for example, makes much of the importance of proper linguistic analysis, but does not discuss the extra hours that would have to be found if such analyses were being done routinely.

[5] But here too there is a need for caution. No linguist should be brought in unless he has first spent some time observing clinical situations, and has learned something of the priorities involved.

grammar, and suggesting, for example, that the complexity of a sentence is in direct proportion to the number of transformations used to generate it (see Yngve 1960, Hayes 1970, Fodor and Garrett 1966, Brown 1973, for discussion). The problems with all these approaches are succinctly summarized by Rees (1971, 287):

> The structural complexity basis therefore appears to offer few substantial guidelines for making decisions in language training. The major problem appears to be that no comprehensive and undisputed analysis of grammatical complexity in relation to sentence processing has been made available. A second problem is that, even should a satisfactory analysis for processing sentences by adult language users become available, applying the results to language training would still involve the untested assumption that the degree of difficulty in sentence production for adults corresponds to the order of difficulty children experience in mastering grammatical constructions.

Current psycholinguistic theory has no coherent explanation for syntactic complexity, and any attempts to assert that some structures are 'more basic' or 'more complex' than others, on intuitive grounds, soon land one in difficulty, if anything other than the most elementary of sentence-building processes are being investigated. Differences of opinion rapidly arise. Menyuk and Looney (1972), for example, assume that appositional structures are more complex than relatives (e.g. *Paul, a Boy Scout, knows how to tie knots* is more complex than *Paul, who is a Boy Scout, knows how to tie knots*), which the present authors find debatable. Lee (1969) sees the order of complexity of *wh*-questions one way; Ingram (1972d) supports a different ordering. Many such examples could be given.[6] Remedial procedures which attempt to operate in this way sometimes begin plausibly enough, but as structures build up, they rapidly become arbitrary, selective, and impressionistic— in a word, pseudoscientific. We were unable to use Conn 1971 after its early stages for this reason, for example. Nor were we able to use those approaches where the measure of structural complexity contradicted developmental ordering, e.g. Morehead and Ingram (1973) found that some transformations are earlier than their base forms (e.g. *he going* before *go*).

Using a linguistic model of structural complexity without a developmental dimension inevitably leads to arbitrariness in assigning values to one's formal categories. Dever's approach, for example, aims to be a purely synchronic descriptive inventory, which does not predict development: 'our attempt to classify was made in terms of the language patterns which occur, not in terms of the development of children' (Dever and Bauman 1971, 15). Each utterance should be capable

---

[6] Lee, in common with most investigators working along these lines, does not explain *why* a structure X is more or less complex than Y, and there thus seems to be a great deal of arbitrary pointing in her method, e.g. *this/that* scores 1, *these/those* scores 4; pronouns score more than nouns (see further Tyack 1972b). Lee and Canter say (1971, 319): 'Within each classification, specific words or structures have been grouped into what is believed to be a general developmental order', on the basis of 'presumably similar degrees of difficulty'—but we are given no rationale, and decisions are often puzzling: e.g. Lee (1969) considers *is going to* as 'more immature' than *will*. Lee (1974) is much more satisfactory in motivating the scoring procedure, and a number of modifications are made.

of being classified at one place in the system: the scale[7] 'requires only that the child be understood—classification then becomes a matter of applying the rules in the scale' (11). His scale, then, 'classifies degrees of approximation to adult English' (17) for clause structure (sentence and phrase structure are to be investigated at a later date). But Dever finds it difficult to match the rank-analyses of the various clauses, and his approach is thus severely limited, to the study of single clauses and clause-types: it cannot be used 'as a scale which indicates generalized development across clauses' (20), which in our opinion is where most of the interest lies.

(b)   A method of ordering structures in terms of their cognitive complexity is also a theoretical possibility. Rees (1971) reviews the main opinions on the relationship between language and thought (that language is central to, incidental to, or parallel to thought) and concludes that 'the literature . . . appears to offer no unified basis' (297). We agree. There is as yet too much controversy for a single viewpoint to suggest itself for reliable widespread clinical application, and there is a tremendous gap between what is known about general cognitive processes and the detail which would need to be established before a reasonably complete remedial programme could be constructed. A few structures have begun to be investigated from the point of view of cognitive/linguistic influence (e.g. Donaldson and Wales 1970), but no overall normative picture has yet emerged.

(c)   It is also possible that structures might be ordered in terms of the perceptual difficulty involved in encoding or decoding them. Certainly Ts are usually well aware of the problems involved due to segmentation, sequencing, category-matching etc. in visual as well as linguistic modes, and there is no denying that a structural grading in these terms would be invaluable. But at present this reasoning is valid on a very small scale, for example in deciding the relative ease of two constructions. Rees thinks that this principle 'suggests useful answers in some cases' (300) and offers 'promising insights into the relative difficulty of grammatical structures upon which the clinician may base his decisions' (302). The technique is rather ad hoc, however, and the notion of perceptual difficulty is still extremely obscure, so that decisions about ordering are inevitably to some extent arbitrary.

(d)   Rees also discusses the possibility that mean length of utterance might provide a basis for structural ordering, and reaches a negative conclusion, as we have already had to do (see chapter 1).

(e)   Nor is there anything to be said about her fifth area, which suggests that structures might be ordered on a dialectal basis—that is, T should provide 'practical information about the structures that the child hears most and with which he will obtain the greatest reinforcement' (302). This is more a general orientation for T than an actual procedure, we feel. Frequency information about structures is difficult to obtain (especially for colloquial speech), and even if norms could be

---

[7] The Indiana Scale of Clausal Development is a classification of the performance patterns of the spontaneous speech of children between 17 and 40 months, using tagmemic clause analysis (cf. Elson & Pickett 1965). On Dever's notion of performance, see further p. 36 below.

established, the relation between frequency and complexity in syntax (as in vocabulary) has hardly been investigated. All that seems certain is that there is no straightforward relationship between them: the most common constructions are not necessarily the least complex, and vice versa.

(*f*) It is Rees's final possibility which, she considers, offers the most grounds for optimism, and which corresponds to the basis on which we ourselves work. This is to order syntactic structures in terms of the normal developmental sequence in the child. Rees finds this 'a useful source of guidelines . . . its application has already proved effective' (302). We would add that, from T's point of view, it is unavoidable:[8] consciously or unconsciously, the analysis of a syntactic disorder inevitably involves a comparison with normal development, and the more the comparative basis can be formalized, the more accurate and constructive one's assessment will be. Rees makes the point: 'The assumption that the normal sequence is somehow the "right" sequence for the language-disordered child to follow has not been proved, but neither has it been seriously challenged' (289). It would be, presumably, if (*i*) some independent measure of complexity could be evolved which produced better results—but we have already seen that this is unlikely in the near future; or if (*ii*) the majority of syntactic disorders were characterized by a predominance of deviant patterns falling quite outside the usage of the normally developing child, and where information about normal syntactic development would accordingly have a limited or negligible explanatory role. To form an opinion on this point, however, one needs to be very clear as to what is meant by the term 'deviant'.

This term is used in the literature on disorders in many different senses, of which three are particularly important: a very general sense, in which deviance subsumes all kinds of linguistic disability (including delay); a more restricted sense, which includes Ps where the range of structures used is comparable to an earlier stage of normal development, but the frequency of use of specific structures falls outside normal expectations; and an extremely narrow sense, in which only certain types of structural abnormality are labelled deviant. Our usage in this book inclines to the latter, which is close to the general sense of the term in linguistics: here, a deviant sentence is one which in some respect does not conform to the grammatical rules of the adult language, e.g. *cat angry are*. In this sense, considerations of frequency of use are not criterial. Some sentences which would be deviant from the viewpoint of adult grammar are however possible when seen in terms of normal child development, e.g. *want horse*, and such constructions would not therefore be considered by us to be deviant, if they occurred as part of P's utterance, but instances of delay. Our final definition of deviance, then, includes only those sentences which would be both structurally inadmissible in the adult grammar, and

---

[8] We therefore find it difficult to accept Lee and Canter's view (1971, 335): 'DSS should not be considered by clinicians as a test of syntactic or morphological development, but rather as a clinical procedure for analysing verbal performance and planning appropriate remedial measures.' But can this distinction really be made? And is it possible to plan without any developmental perspective at all? If not, then it is important that this be made explicit.

not part of the expected grammatical development of normal children (insofar as this can be established by reference to the language acquisition literature). For example, if P said *cat the*, this would be considered deviant on the grounds that an adult grammar would reject this construction and that this pattern has not been noted as a regular feature of normal language development. It is obvious that this definition is not as precise as we would like it to be: there are too many gaps in the research literature for us to be sure sometimes whether a construction is deviant or not; also, we must not underestimate the extent to which problems of grammatical acceptability (see Quirk and Svartvik 1966) cause difficulties. But as an operational tool, we have found this notion of deviance useful. It must however be clearly distinguished from other senses found in the literature on syntactic remediation, e.g. Leonard (1972), who emphasizes the importance of different frequencies of use as a criterion of deviance v. delay. Our assessment procedure focuses at present only on the *qualitative* range of structures used by P. We only ask the question whether, regardless of frequency, the structures used are possible adult or expected normal child sentences. If the answer is no, this is then a deviant sentence for us. If the answer is yes, it is nondeviant—though it may still be deviant, in a frequency sense, for other scholars, e.g. Menyuk 1964, Leonard 1972.

This does not commit us to the view that Ps with no deviant sentences are 'delayed' in any simple sense. The concept of delay is at least as complicated as that of deviance. Some Ps are delayed quite literally, in the sense that their speech is a replica of their juniors; some are delayed in certain structural respects only; some are delayed solely in terms of frequency of use. Most definitions of delay contain a number of criteria, therefore: e.g. Ingram (1972a, 89) and Morehead and Ingram (1973, 340) conclude that disorder is a function of slower onset of time of appearance of a structure, its less frequent and less creative use, and its slower acquisition time. Comparison of different studies is complicated also by problems of selecting and matching the groups of children being compared, and also by the use of linguistic models which focus on different features of syntactic structure. We nonetheless have the impression that most of the studies of the nature of a language disorder conclude that deviant sentences in our sense are relatively uncommon with children, and only slightly more of a problem with adults. It would therefore seem to follow that the scope of a remediation procedure can be modelled on the range of structures present at the various stages of child development, up to and including adult use. Dever, for example, says (1973, 3): 'a description of what normal children do while learning their native language will constitute an adequate statement of the sequence of goal behaviors of a language teaching program.' And in essence, this view seems to be widely supported: see, for example, Lenneberg *et al.* 1964, Lackner 1968, Miller and Yoder 1974, Rosenberg 1973, Pressnell 1973.

To use a normal developmental hypothesis as a basis for ordering structure has much to commend it, particularly as its empirical support is based on the fewest possible assumptions about complexity of language processing. It is important to realize that claims made on this basis say *nothing* about complexity, of any kind. Just because a child learns to use structure X before structure Y does not necessarily mean that X is less complex than Y. All sorts of other factors—of which motivation is probably the most important—interfere with such a judgement. All that can be said is that if it can be shown that there is a normal (i.e. natural) developmental path for syntax, this is itself a motivation for developing a remedial procedure in its terms. How the procedure is to be implemented is of course a separate issue for T. We are not saying that the disordered child must be treated as if he were normal, e.g. in terms of the amount of routine correction of 'mistakes' which he might be given. Specific therapeutic procedures will be necessary. But we are saying that the grounds for selecting the structures to teach, the specification of the teaching goals, and the entire process of assessment can usefully be done within a framework geared to a normal developmental scale. And this is what we shall present in chapter 4.

Before going on to this, however, there are a few other points which need to be made about the use of such a scale. To begin with, it must be made clear that, in the present state of knowledge, we see this scale rather as the 'least unsatisfactory' method of all that have been suggested. The scale of chapter 4 is a synthesis of what is known about developing syntax in children. There are, consequently, many gaps. But while language acquisition studies of syntax have a great way to go before anything like a complete account emerges, we feel that enough information is available now to enable the outline of a remedial approach to be drawn with confidence, and for many areas of detail to be filled in. For assessment, as we shall see, it is the well-defined and comprehensive outline which is all-important—the notion of a 'syntactic profile'—and here there is enough data on which to build.

A related point is that we maintain that any linguistic remediation procedure based on developmental norms that does not attempt to correlate its structural stages with chronological age is shirking the main issue. Chronological age is the one thing that impinges on T at all stages, and it cannot be ignored. That a child is not 'up to his age' is the basis for most parental concern, and enters into the decision-making process at all stages—referral, assessment, and release. (It is less important in deciding upon the path through a remedial procedure.) If, then, a syntactic procedure is to be of use to teachers, educational psychologists, clinicians, and others, information about chronological norms must be included. Popular and professional intuitions make the correlation: it is the job of the linguist to explicate it. On reading the language acquisition literature, however, the most noticeable thing is the way in which writers *avoid* the issue of chronological norms. Thus Brown (1973) summarizes a decade of attitudes when he writes: 'Though the order of acquisition of linguistic knowledge will prove to be approximately invariant across children learning one language and, at a higher level of abstraction, across children learning any language, the rate of progression will vary radically among children' (1973, 408). We accept that information about ordering is a valuable means of grading structures for therapeutic intervention, and also as a research tool, but by itself it is of restricted value in assessing the kinds and degree of severity of child language disorders—particularly as most Ps are evidencing some stage of language delay. *How great* is the delay is the persistent question. This is the information that parents want to have, and no amount of talking around the subject in terms of 'syntactic relativity' avoids this. So the question is, Is the variability in rate of syntactic development pointed out by Brown and others *sufficiently great* for the whole notion of chronological age norms to be thrown out altogether? This would seem to be an absurd conclusion. All of us have clear intuitions about norms of fluency and expressiveness in young children.[9] We are aware that some children are 'very advanced for their age' and that others are not very talkative. In the light of this, it is likely that the emphasis on rate variability in the literature is at least partly due to analysis so far having been restricted to intensive studies of a very few children: differences between individuals become more marked under the microscope, and as a larger range of children come to be studied, we predict that striking similarities in rate of acquisition of structures will emerge. When one compares the empirical findings of language-acquisition studies, in fact, it is surprising how similar dates of predominant development of the various syntactic structures turn out to be. Onset time and hypothetical acquisition time may indeed vary, but means display a remarkable correspondence. For example, every reference we have ever seen to the emergence of two-element sentences (e.g. *daddy see*) cites the age-range of between 18 months and 2 years. But even when we look at more specific features, such as question-words, specific word-order patterns, modal verbs, and so on, we find that their dates of emergence with a productive role generally cluster within a period of about 6 months. A 6-month variability (± 3 months around a mean date of emergence) may seem vague to the theoretical psycholinguist, but it is an extremely precise indication in remedial work, compared with the impressionism and absence of quantitative measures of syntactic development that is apparent.

Lastly in this section, it might be objected that, while structural grading based on norms of child development may be satisfactory for remedial work with children, this principle is inapplicable for work with adults. As will be clear from chapter 8, we have not found it so. If an adult displays a disorder capable of being defined in syntactic terms, we find that the assessment of the disability, and its subsequent remediation, can be carried out using exactly the same scale of syntactic development as we use with children. There are certain differences in the use of the syntactic procedure, which will be referred to in later chapters, but these are outweighed by the similarities. Myerson and Goodglass seem to have reached a similar conclusion (1972, 41): 'Taking samples from patients at various severity levels is analogous to examining speech samples from children at different ages.' This is not to subscribe to a general regression hypothesis for adult dysphasics, i.e. the structures the adult will have learned last will be lost first. We do not know whether this is a defensible hypothesis, evidence of gradual loss of structure being

---

[9] We know of no systematic work rating people's abilities to make consistent judgements of such levels of ability—whether this varies between mothers, fathers, nurses, linguists etc.—but we have no doubt that such abilities exist and will provide part of the evidence for descriptive decisions. Naturally, any well-developed theory of syntactic ability will have to take into account the variables of socioeconomic background, sex, intelligence, health, and so on; but we do not wish to underestimate the ability of (especially) the mother to take these variations unconsciously into account in judging the level of linguistic development of the child.

almost impossible to find, in view of the nature of the traumas involved; but there is certainly evidence against it: e.g. Myerson and Goodglass show that optional adverbials are quite well retained in their Ps, though these are learned relatively late, whereas some quite basic structural relationships had disappeared. Moreover, we do not know—nor, in the present state of knowledge, see a way of knowing— to what extent a disorder is a matter of competence or performance, i.e. whether the underlying system is lost, or is there but unable to get out. The latter view seems the more likely (as argued by Weigl and Bierwisch 1970, Sefer and Shaw 1972 etc.), in view of the way in which most Ps we have encountered respond to therapy, but this is speculation. In other words, we have no *theoretical* reasons for using the child development scale in relation to adults. Our arguments are pragmatic: we have found no viable alternative, and by using it satisfactory progress in Ps' use of syntax has been achieved.

In this chapter we have discussed some of the criteria we use in order to evaluate remedial procedures in syntax, and which we have tried to follow in developing our own. We present our procedure in chapter 5. Before doing this, however, we must outline the descriptive and developmental frameworks we shall need to use in order to meet the demands made above. Chapter 3 describes the system of syntactic description, chapter 4 the stages of syntactic development in children.

3

The syntactic framework of description

It is clear from the preceding chapters that a number of different linguistic approaches have been applied to the analysis of language disorder. It would be unwise, however, to assume that all of these approaches, and the models they use, are equally easy to work with in the study of a given applied language field. As far as the subject of language disability is concerned, this is certainly not so. We have looked at this field from many positions within linguistics, and find that whereas all theories are in principle capable of describing the character of a language disorder, certain approaches are much more immediately illuminating and easier to work with than others. Before giving a detailed description of the approach we have chosen to work with ourselves, therefore, it may be helpful to outline the main reasons which led to our choice.[1]

For historical reasons, in this area of evaluation, the first question that has to be posed is how usable is the transformational-generative (TG) approach in investigating these matters. It would seem sensible to open any discussion with reference to this view, as owing to the influence of TG theory over the past twenty years, many Ts, having learned something of it, find that their first question is pre-empted by the climate of opinion, and they find themselves asking 'Do I use TG in my work or not?' And certainly, there have been a number of attempts to use TG in one or other of its forms in the study of language disability, e.g. Braun and Klassen 1971, Wachal and Spreen 1970, Spreen and Wachal 1973, Muma 1971, Hass and Wepman 1969, Leonard 1972, Menyuk and Looney 1972, Davis 1973, Morehead and Ingram 1973. Some indeed have claimed that only TG is worth using, e.g. Rosenberg, cited in Dever and Bauman 1971. In addition, there are a number of approaches which incorporate aspects of TG into their work, e.g. Myerson and Goodglass 1972, Miller and Yoder 1974. Lee's work (see above) claims to be transformational in principle, but it is hardly that, as the approach is basically a selection of hierarchically organized structural features, largely operating at phrase level (cf. below), with some analyses of generative origin, especially of the verb phrase, introduced. We ought also to add that frequently work in language disorders seriously misunderstands the nature of a generative grammar, usually by confusing the notions of competence and performance. We have often encountered Ts who see TG as a language-teaching kit, and who think

[1] Until theoretically sound evaluation procedures for grammars are devised, decisions about the choice of grammar to use must inevitably be pragmatic and to some degree personal. The following discussion of alternatives very much reflects these considerations.

that what is being advised is to teach a child phrase-structure rules first, and transformations later!

There is, then, a great deal of interest in the application of TG in this field, but the results have been disappointing. The main reason is that the most important studies have shown that the salient differentiating features are precisely those *not* readily describable in terms of the most important characteristics of the TG model. The set of transformations, for example, as defined by Chomsky (1957a or 1965) have turned out to be singularly undiscriminating. The syntactic features which most directly distinguish the various kinds of ability which we want to characterize emerge as being sentence construction types (i.e. patterns of Subject, Verb, Object etc.; see below), which TG on the whole pays little attention to, and which other models treat in a much more direct way. Muma (1971), for example, uses a 1957 model of TG to analyse 13 fluent and 13 nonfluent 4-year-olds, and finds no difference in the overall number of transformations per sentence.[2] He ends his paper suggesting that alternative approaches might be better, especially in so far as they would analyse performance and pay attention to sentence-types (which *did* differentiate his groups). Morehead and Ingram (1973) use Rosenbaum 1967 to do a complex transformational analysis of 15 normal and 15 deviant children, selected to represent the five linguistic levels previously determined by Brown (1973). In order to establish the nature of the deficit in the deviant group, they examine a large number of transformations, but find little difference in either the organization or the occurrence of transformational features at a given linguistic level: 'there is considerable similarity in the transformational development of both groups across the five levels of linguistic development' (337). On the other hand, information about constructional type does have value: 'deviant children appear to be significantly restricted in their ability to develop and select grammatical and semantic features which allow existent and new major lexical categories to be assigned to larger sets of syntactic frames' (343). Likewise, Morehead (1972) concludes that comparison in terms of constructional type is 'the only meaningful difference' (4) between normal and deviant children: 'the deviant child's deficit lies not in his ability to develop base aspects of grammar but rather in his ability to develop additional terms and the relations in which to use those terms' (5). (See also Lozar *et al.* (1973, 29), who found sentence-level units to be the only significant differences between retarded and normal children's syntax.)

The main evidence for the difficulty in using the TG model, then, comes from those who have tried to work with it systematically, and it is interesting that, in their search for alternatives, their suggestions all point in the same direction. This direction is precisely that concluded by Longhurst and Schrandt (1973) who, having compared four measures of analysis, say: 'A renewed interest in basic structural linguistic concepts could prove valuable to the assessment of language development in children. This interest should be focussed on such topics as analysing how verbs develop at six-month intervals or how the various "features of arrangement"

---

[2] There was some suggestion that the nonfluent children used more single-base and less double-base transformations, in fact, but this was not felt to be significant.

develop . . .' (248). This is exactly our position, as will be described below. But it is worth pointing out that a structuralist orientation does not preclude our using certain transformational notions; indeed, the grammatical framework on which our approach is based frequently incorporates them, especially in describing the output of older children and adults. But we have never found an analysis in transformational terms to be useful for more than a small part of the overall picture.

We do not wish to speculate at length about the reason for this, but if anything it is likely to be due to the difficulty in working with any model based on the fundamental insight of the TG approach, namely, that language can be seen as a single system of generative process. A TG grammar works by assigning the same initial analysis to all the sentences of a language (of which the earliest and most well-known formulation was S → NP + VP, i.e. 'Rewrite Sentence as Noun Phrase plus Verb Phrase'), and then progressively expanding, removing, or reordering the various constituents by a sequence of rules so that one finally emerges with a detailed specification of the structural features of a sentence. Working backwards, this means that, given the structural analysis of any sentence in the language, it is possible to follow the reasoning which led to this analysis being assigned by examining the various stages in its derivation; ultimately, the sentence will be shown to have been generated from the initial rule, and, by implication, related to all other sentences in the language. The possibility of attributing psychological reality to these underlying, or 'deep' structures has then often been claimed. Now this kind of approach has some plausibility in normal adult language studies, particularly when it succeeds in explicitly and formally relating sentences which we intuitively feel to be closely related, but which traditional approaches to grammar would have kept apart or ignored. But in studies of abnormality, where the intuitions of the 'native speakers' are fragile and indeterminate, to say the least, the justification for assigning a particular derivation to a sentence becomes extremely difficult, and is usually arbitrary and implausible. We would want to argue that a remediation procedure in particular should make the fewest possible assumptions about the nature of the mental reality underlying speech, and concentrate instead on an exhaustive account of the characteristics of the speech actually produced by P and T. While accepting that there may be a case for the empirical study of competence in (Chomsky's sense) in normal adults, we find this notion, its formalization in transformational terms, and the more powerful notion of innate structure, which is usually associated with it, extremely difficult to work with in the young child, and impossible to work with in evaluating disorders in either children or adults. In such cases the distinction between competence and performance becomes an unreal issue, and the linguist is forced to rely on a minute analysis of whatever speech he can manage to elicit, in order to provide a basis for therapeutic intervention. (This means, among other things, paying particular attention to the intonational, pausal and other prosodic features of both P and T, which we have found to play an influential role in both assessment and remediation, as is illustrated in chapters 7 and 8.) Scepticism about competence models, and emphasis upon performance data, is in fact increasing in the field of language disturbance, e.g. Engler et al. (1973, 196) conclude: 'the task is to identify and count constructions in speech samples of real clients rather than to ponder the competence of the "ideal speaker" ' (and see also Morehead and Ingram 1973, Lee and Canter 1971). Two points should be noted here. Firstly, the scepticism is being directed at a specifically Chomskyan notion of a competence involving deep structures (which are only one way of formalizing our intuitions.) Everyone must be interested in making claims about the underlying system of the child's language ability; it is the way of approaching this which is under attack. Secondly, one wants to argue for a proper *emphasis* on performance, not an exclusive concentration on it, as again it is the systematic use of language that counts in any assessment. Confusion over both these points underlies aspects of the discussion in Dever and Bauman 1971, for example. They claim that their approach, derived from tagmemics, is a grammar of performance—but this is not so. Their grammar does pay more attention to features of performance than TG, it is true, but that does not make it a performance grammar in any strict sense nor do the authors want it to be. That their real concern is with the underlying system emerges clearly at many points, e.g. 'the single most important defining feature of any clause is the presence or *potential presence* of a verbal element as one of the nuclear tagmemes' (17, our italics), or again, and more explicitly: 'In their abstract form any utterance rule could become confused with almost any other rule. Therefore, use of the scale relies very heavily on the knowledge that each native speaker has of his language for determining whether a clause is to be classified as being declarative, question or imperative' (20), and 'there seems to be no efficient way to define these categories except to say that every native speaker of English knows when a clause is to be classified as one of the three' (17).[3]

There is also a pragmatic difficulty which accounts for our disillusionment with TG. This arises out of the rapid development of that theory since 1957. This has caused inevitable difficulties in all applied fields, as practitioners continually run the risk of being told that their conception of syntactic theory is out of date (even if, sometimes, by only 6 months or a year!). Much of the early work in clinical applications, which tried, for example, to analyse disorders in terms of kernel and nonkernel sentences, would now presumably be dismissed as ill-conceived theoretically (e.g. Lee and Canter's use of the 1957 analysis of the verb phrase; or Davis (1973), who distinguishes kernel sentences, minor transformations (e.g. inflections and function words), and major transformations (change of sentence type)). So would Hass and Wepman's views (1969), e.g. 'It now makes sense to consider deep structure as forming the same sort of borderline between syntactic and semantic processes as surface structure forms between syntactic and phonological ones' (304). The differences between the various positions are by no means trivial, and make it extremely difficult to compare the results of people working with different models, e.g. Muma, and Morehead and Ingram. And if the inquirer

[3] Dever and Bauman seem to have underestimated the role of 'surface' structure (continuing the generative metaphor) in reaching this conclusion, in fact. After all, if the categories are being used systematically by native speakers, there *must* be a basis for this. Intonation in particular is a factor, as they recognize, but while they accept that their rules vary 'only in the intonational envelope at times', this is nonetheless 'a feature which is not formally expressed in the scale' (20).

after syntactic truth seeks to avoid the theoretical disputes of the early TG models by turning to the more recent work, there is no solace: controversy and change abound still, and the emphasis is increasingly less syntactic and more semantic, with few frameworks of any descriptive range and depth of detail emerging. Until such time, then, as successful studies of disorders are made within the TG tradition, we prefer to develop our syntactic procedures using other sources.

But which? The safest course of action would seem to be to choose a syntactic framework that has been fairly stable over a period of time, and which is sufficiently flexible to permit the use where necessary of insights from the recent approaches. The obvious place to turn is to the general tradition of structuralist linguistics in the United States and Europe, which was the dominant mode of syntactic investigation in the period preceding Chomsky (late 1940s to mid-1950s). Many distinct theoretical approaches developed out of this tradition—perhaps the most well known being those of K. L. Pike ('tagmemic theory') in the USA, and M. A. K. Halliday (first 'scale-and-category grammar', later 'systemic grammar') in Great Britain. Richard Dever and his associates are currently working on the clinical application of tagmemic theory (see Dever 1972a, 1973, Dever and Bauman 1971, and above, p. 23). We know of no work being done using a Hallidayan framework. There is however a certain amount of published material which does not aim to start from a coherent general linguistic theory, but works within an ad hoc structuralist framework, e.g. Engler *et al.* 1973, Conn 1971, Thomas 1971, Morehead and Johnson 1972, Ingram 1972b, Foster *et al.* n.d., Williams and Naremore 1969, Reynell 1969. Most of this, we find, is clinically highly relevant. At times, indeed, the similarity to our own approach is so close as to be almost embarrassing! Engler *et al.*, for example, have developed a technique they call the 'linguistic analysis of speech samples' (LASS), which aims to produce a 'diagnostic profile' of spontaneous speech, is eclectic (incorporating ideas from tagmemics, immediate constituent analysis, and TG), and contrastive (samples are compared with the language of the clinician or with other children of the same age and development). They also pay particular attention to the role of the verb and its classification (though Longhurst and Schrandt (1973, 246) claim that this could not distinguish the two children in their study). The parallelism with chapter 5 below is remarkable. There are however important differences. Perhaps the most far-reaching is that Engler *et al.* do not make any explicit connection with an established grammatical tradition; as already mentioned, their article presents a highly simplified and schematic account of English syntax, with no criteria or discussion to help T handle the problem areas of analysis. Also, because it is not geared to any set of developmental norms, their analysis is burdened with a number of descriptive categories which we have found to be unnecessary. But the general emphasis in their approach (as well as that found in the other references above) is correct, in our view, and we have been much reassured in our own work by becoming aware of these parallels.

In our work, then, we have tried to make use of a descriptive framework which reflects the above emphases, and which is easily and directly applicable to the study of grammatical disability. We have chosen to work with a framework based on a recently published approach entitled *A grammar of contemporary English* (Quirk *et al.* 1972). An abridged version is available under the title *A university grammar of English* (Quirk and Greenbaum 1973), and as this is in many ways a more practicable manual for Ts to use, we add references to this (*UGE*) as well as to the main grammar (*GCE*) in the description below.

This grammar is the culmination of a decade of work directed by the first author at University College London, where the Survey of English Usage has been in progress since 1960. This survey has as its aim the full description of actual educated spoken and written usage, which would constitute a 'descriptive register' capable of acting as a basis for realistic handbooks of English grammar—in much the same way as the great *New English Dictionary* has acted as a sourcebook for many smaller 'practical' dictionaries of the language. *GCE* is the first major synthesis to be based on this data, and in its empirical emphasis one finds in its pages much more information about the norms of spoken syntax than was presented in the earlier grammatical handbooks of English (such as those of Jespersen, Poutsma, Curme and Kruisinga), within whose general tradition this book falls. Most of *GCE*'s examples are taken or adapted from the collections of data constituting the survey, or from the acceptability experiments which were associated with it (see e.g. Quirk and Svartvik 1966). The emphasis on intonation in relation to syntax is a major feature, as is its stylistic range. The scope is 'the grammar of Educated English current in the second half of the twentieth century in the world's major English-speaking communities' (Preface), emphasizing the 'common core' of the English of serious exposition, but by no means ignoring the restricted styles. It gives clear recognition to the existence of variations in use within the language— to such differences as distinguish speech from writing, formal from informal, American from British. There is no condemnation or neglect of minority usage in this book: it is, above all, a democratic grammar.

GCE is intended to function as a *reference grammar*, that is, as a handbook which can be consulted in order to find out the facts of usage in the language, the regular patterns that constitute the grammatical structure as well as the exceptions-to-rules and problem cases. It is not the kind of grammar which aims to present a coherent theory of language structure as a whole (including phonology and semantics) or to maintain a particular theoretical viewpoint that is generally applicable to languages other than English—such as one finds in Chomsky 1957a. There is a minimum of theoretical exposition, or discussion of how the facts of English motivate one to see grammar in one way rather than another. As far as is feasible, the patterns of structure are allowed to speak for themselves, with the emphasis away from general theoretical implications. And conversely, whenever a feature from some linguistic model seems illuminating for an area of English syntax, it is used. This is not a transformational grammar in principle, for instance, but the use of transformations is to be found at various points throughout the book. To some theoretical linguists, of course, this kind of approach to a language is in principle unsatisfactory, as for them the facts of English are of interest only insofar as they shed light on more general processes of language formation, and to propose an 'eclectic' account of a language (i.e. one which brings together different theoretical traditions and assumptions without explicitly relating them into a fresh coherent theory) is to bypass major difficulties. But for those interested solely in establishing and interrelating the patterns of structure of English as an end in itself, the lack of any such general theoretical foundation will not be crucial. Of far greater importance will be the comprehensiveness of its lists of features (e.g. irregular nouns, types of sentence connecter) and the clarity of its descriptive apparatus and terminology; and in both these respects we have found *GCE* to provide less of a problem than the other approaches with which we are familiar. Most of the terms in it will in fact be recognizable to anyone brought up on a diet of school grammar (though of course some of the definitions have had to be modified, in the interests of consistency and precision).

Terminology and notation from a theoretical point of view, are of course of relatively trivial concern (but cf. Lyons 1963, 5). What you call an entity is unimportant, compared with the reasoning and criteria which led you to identify that entity in the first place. But in applied fields of study, terminology takes on an importance far out of proportion to this, and rightly so. It is arrogant of the theoretical linguist to present a linguistic technique for practical use by non-linguists without making some effort to bridge the gap from his side between his own technicality and the tradition of the nonspecialist, and one way of doing this is by the deliberate use of familiar terms. People seem more ready to take to familiar terms which have been given new definitions than to accept new terms which go with such definitions, particularly when—as is normal these days—the new terms are not isolates, but complex sets of terminology and notation, which must be mastered all at once, as a system, if any of it is to be learned at all. It is essentially a question of basic motivation, in our view. People seem to be more motivated to master and use a technique if they are not put off by its appearance—and no amount of reasoning from the theoretician that 'appearances don't matter' seems able to alter this fact of busy clinical and teaching life. It therefore ranks high in our list of syntactic priorities. We are, after all, only interested in developing a syntactic procedure if it stands a reasonable chance of being used.

The main reasons why we use this approach, then, are twofold. Firstly, it provides as comprehensive a description of contemporary English (at least of its educated 'core') as the present state of knowledge allows, and this ensures that the vast majority of the structures used by P or T will be given some treatment. Secondly, we have found that the organization of this grammar in terms of *levels* (of sentence, clause, phrase, word), its emphasis at clause level on the functional relationships between the various elements of structure, and its account of the role of intonation in English syntax, permits a direct and economical description of the data of syntactic disability, and correlates well with T's intuitions about syntactic patterning (see further chapter 6 for discussion of disorders located primarily at clause level, phrase level etc.).

Before introducing the range of structures from *GCE* which acts as our syntactic framework, it is perhaps worth outlining the organization of the book as a whole, and noting any major departures we make from it. We shall be cross-referring to the various sections of the book during our own exposition below; consequently it would seem useful to present some overall conspectus of its contents. (Alternatively, this summary may be read *after* our own exposition, in which case the reader is advised to continue now on p. 42.)

Chapter 1 provides a general discussion of the contemporary importance of the English language, of the main senses of the term 'grammar' and its relationship to other aspects of linguistic structure, and reviews the main varieties of the language that any description has to distinguish—notions of standard, dialect, specialist styles etc. For those who have read little in linguistic approaches to the description of English, it provides a useful perspective.

Chapter 2 gives a preliminary view of the sentence. It introduces and illustrates the main elements of sentence structure (Subject, Object etc.), and outlines the basic types of sentence, and the major transformational processes which operate on them (question, negation, exclamation, passive and imperative). The chapter also contains a discussion of parts of speech and some of the limitations of this notion. In other words, it provides an overview of the grammar as a whole, and should be read first, in any systematic approach to this book.[4]

Chapters 3 to 6 study the special characteristics of the various elements of sentence structure. Chapter 3 presents the grammar and semantics of the verb phrase; chapter 4 examines the basic structure of the noun phrase, and related items; chapter 5 studies adjectives and adverbs; and chapter 6 is devoted to the relations expressed by prepositions and prepositional phrases.

Chapter 3 begins by classifying the various classes of verb operating in the verb phrase, makes the distinction between finite and non-finite verb phrases and presents the types of each, and summarizes the characteristics of auxiliary verbs. The tense and aspect forms of the verb are then outlined, followed by the meanings of the modal auxiliaries. The chapter concludes with a comprehensive classification of regular and irregular lexical verbs.

Chapter 4 begins with a classification of nouns, with particular reference to the division in terms of proper/common and mass/count. The determiner system is then outlined, with its main subdivisions into predeterminers, ordinals and quantifiers. The role of the articles in specifying the reference of nouns is then discussed, and followed by a classification of noun types in terms of number, gender and case. The chapter concludes with a classification of pronouns into their many different types. We have followed this chapter fairly closely, as many of the frequently occurring problems of syntactic analysis in English involve items

---

[4] It should be noted that certain distinctions are made in the description of the verb phrase which we have not found it necessary to incorporate in our own initial analyses, namely the distinctions between 'static' and 'dynamic' verbs, between 'operator' and 'auxiliary', and the verb category labels 'ditransitive' etc.

dealt with here—in particular, items (e.g. *enough, one, many, all*) that have no single grammatical role, but function in a range of structures.[5]

Chapter 5 examines the characteristics of adjectives, especially in relation to adverbs, nouns and participles, and describes their use in attributive (premodifying) and predicative (complement) functions. Three classes of adverb are then distinguished—adjuncts (integrated within the clause), and disjuncts/conjuncts (which have an evaluative or connecting function). We do not use these distinctions in our approach. Types of adverbial intensifier are then presented, and the chapter concludes with the analysis of comparison.

Chapter 6 is largely devoted to the grammar and semantics of prepositions—of place, time, cause etc. It is preceded by an outline of some of the restrictions on their use, an analysis of 'complex' prepositions, and the distinction between prepositions and prepositional adverbs. Other aspects of prepositional phrases, such as their position and internal modification, are then discussed.

Chapter 7 then takes up the study of simple sentence structure from chapter 2, and the main transformational processes, insofar as they affect all elements except the adverbial. This is the most important chapter, as it relates closely to the basis of our approach. It begins by distinguishing the seven main clause types built up out of different combinations of elements, and proceeds to detail the semantic functions of the subject and object elements of structure, and thence to a discussion of concord between the elements. The vocative is given separate discussion. The various processes of negation within the sentence are then distinguished, followed by a description of the formal features of statement, question, command and exclamation. A separate category of echo-utterances is established. The chapter concludes with a brief account of types of formulaic utterance etc.—what our approach subsumes under the heading of Minor sentences (not a *GCE* term). Apart from this, we follow the analysis in this chapter quite closely.

Chapter 8 is entirely devoted to the detailed discussion of types of adverbials, and the reasons for distinguishing adjuncts, disjuncts and conjuncts, thus amplifying the relevant part of chapter 5. The subdivisions are largely based on semantic considerations, and we have not incorporated them into our own approach.

Chapter 9 presents a description of ellipsis, coordination and apposition—three ways of expanding or modifying the basic patterns of sentence structure. A wide range of types of elliptical construction is described. The distinction between coordination and subordination is made in clause linkage, and the types of coordination illustrated, particular reference being made to the possibilities of ellipsis. The types of phrasal coordination are then outlined, again with reference

[5] Our only modification is in the use of the term 'Initiator' for 'Predeterminer', and the general label 'Adjectival' to subsume Ordinals and Quantifiers as well as more central kinds of adjective.

to ellipsis, and this leads into a description of types of apposition, and related kinds of connectivity. We do not in our approach enter into detail under any of these headings, but we do make use of all the major distinctions.

Chapter 10 follows naturally from this, dealing with the links which relate one sentence to another. Semantic, lexical and syntactic means of sentence connection are distinguished, and the syntactic devices described in detail: time and place relaters, logical connecters, substitution forms, features of discourse reference, comparison, ellipsis and structural parallelism. Our own approach is largely within the sentence, but insofar as sentence sequences are taken into account, we follow the distinctions made in this chapter fairly closely.

Chapter 11 takes up the distinction between coordination and subordination, and examines how one or more sentences may be subordinated within another. Three types of dependent clause are established on structural grounds—finite, nonfinite, and verbless; the formal indicators of subordination are classified; and the range of functions of these clauses in the sentence presented—noun, adverbial, relative, comparative and comment. The chapter concludes with the rules for the use of the verb phrase in dependent clauses, and the distinction between direct and indirect speech.

Chapter 12 follows up chapter 3 by looking more closely at the types of verb phrase in relation to the complement structures which may follow them. It deals with the distinction between active and passive voice, between phrasal and pre-positional verbs, and classifies the various types of complement structures. This is a complex area of English syntax, and we make use of only the most general categories in our approach.

Chapter 13 follows up chapter 4 in exploring the full complexity that it is possible for the noun phrase to have by taking within itself the structures separately examined in earlier chapters. The distinctions between head, premodification and postmodification, and between restrictive and nonrestrictive kinds of modification are introduced.

Chapter 14 deals with the way in which the various parts of the sentence can be arranged to have different kinds of prominence, such as contrast, emphasis and reinforcement. Constructions using *it* and *there* are described, along with variations in word order and intonation.

There are three *Appendices*: on word formation; stress, rhythm and intonation; and punctuation.

Our syntactic description

The salient features of the method of syntactic analysis we use may be summarized as follows.

It is normal to begin syntactic analysis with the *Sentence*.[6] There are three main tasks: (*a*) to identify the sentences in the data; (*b*) to analyse their structure and function; and (*c*) to analyse the way they combine into 'connected speech'.

A   Identification

In writing, this is usually no problem: sentences begin with capital letters and end with one of a small set of concluding punctuation marks (full stop, question mark etc.). In speech, there is sometimes a problem: falling intonation tones and the presence of a pause *may* mark a sentence-ending, but they do not always, and sometimes it is difficult to say if you have come to the end of a sentence or not. For example, in writing, these two utterances have a different structure:

> I'm coming at three. And Mary's coming at four.
> I'm coming at three; and Mary's coming at four.

But in speech, these may sound exactly the same, and the analyst does not know whether to count one sentence or two. Usually not more than about 5 per cent of normal adult data causes problems of this kind. Problems of sentence identification become greater in disordered speech and in child language, however, and debatable cases must be classified separately (see further chapter 5).

B   Analysis of sentence structure

Let us assume, then, that we have before us a list of sentences whose identification has not been problematic. What are the most important features of structure to be singled out?

It is not possible to summarize all the facts of sentence structure in a single statement. The idea of 'complex' sentence structure is not a single, simple notion, for instance, as the complexity distributes itself around the sentence in various ways: a sentence may be complex when looked at from one point of view, but simple when seen from another. The idea that sentences have different 'levels' of structure, each of which has its own kind of patterning, is central to our description of syntax.

An analysis, also, must begin with the most general and abstract facts about sentence structure, before proceeding systematically to the more detailed points which have to be made.

In this approach, three main levels of sentence structure are recognized:[7]

(*i*)   patterns of sentence and clause structure
(*ii*) patterns of phrase structure
(*iii*) patterns of word structure.

In addition, there is (*iv*), the patterns of sentence connection, mentioned above.

---

[6] For alternative views, using the morpheme, word etc., see Crystal 1971a.
[7] These levels are also used by Dever and his colleagues (see 1971, 1973).

C Patterns of sentence and clause structure

1 It is helpful to begin by making a very broad twofold classification of all the sentences in the data, distinguishing MAJOR and MINOR sentences.

2 Major sentences, essentially, have a Subject–Predicate structure. Minor sentences do not.

Major sentences are like:

> *John kicked the ball.*
> *We're going to the match at three o'clock.*
> *All the children came in when the teacher called.*
> *Are you happy in your work?*

Minor sentences are like:

> *Yes. Oh! Hello.*
> *First come, first served.*

(These are obviously going to be particularly common in informal speech.)

3 We must now state the range of patterns which fall under these two headings. As most of the data will probably be major sentences, this seems the obvious place to start.

Major sentences may be SIMPLE or MULTIPLE. A simple major sentence is one with just a single CLAUSE. A multiple major sentence contains a sequence of clauses, which are linked in various ways. A simple sentence would be:

> *John kicked the ball.*

A multiple sentence would be:

> *John kicked the ball and then he fell over.*
> *John kicked the ball because he wanted to.*

So what is a clause?[8]

4 Clauses are of various kinds, but their structure is always defined with reference to a small, fixed set of elements, such as 'subject', 'verb', 'object'. Exactly how many there are will be stated below. But one of them is central: the VERB. The verb is the most important part of a clause, because it determines most of the patterns which are allowed to appear in the rest of the sentence.

It is always possible to tell what the verb is in a clause, as it is the word which belongs to a set of forms which vary in a predictable way: they vary for tense (e.g. *I walk/I walked*); they have different participle forms (*walking/walked*); and they can be used immediately after the set of seven words called personal pronouns

---

[8] This emphasis on the clause is at the core of Dever's work, especially the Indiana Scale of Clausal Development (see Dever and Bauman 1971, Dever 1973) based on tagmemic analysis (Elson and Pickett 1965).

(*I, you, he, she, it, we, they*). Sometimes more than one word joins together to act as verb, as in *He **is coming*** (see further below).

5   In a clause, the verb (V) usually has a SUBJECT (S). In its simplest form, then, the major sentence is of the pattern SV, e.g.

> *John's coming.*
> *It's raining.*
> *The big boys laughed.*

(Whenever a verb could be used like this, without any further structure following it, it would be called an 'intransitive' verb, in traditional grammar.)

The only important case where a major sentence verb may appear without a subject is in commands (though even here, a subject is often present), e.g.

> *Go! Look! You go! All you boys look!*

6   Verbs determine the structure of the rest of the clause in various ways. Some verbs, firstly, govern an OBJECT (O), as in:

> *I kicked him.   The big boys saw the little girls.*
> S   V   O   S   V   O

This is usually referred to as the 'direct' object.

Other verbs may govern two objects—an indirect (i), as well as a direct (d) object, as in:

> *I gave a book to the girl.*   or,   *I gave the girl a book.*
> S V O_d O_i S V O_i O_d

7   Some verbs may govern a COMPLEMENT (C)—a word or phrase which specifies something further about the subject or object, e.g.

> *He is a man.   The boy seems ready.   They made him a doctor.*
> S V C   S   V   C   S   V   O   C
> (i.e. the ready boy)   (i.e. He *is* the doctor)

The verb *to be* when used as the sole verb is usually referred to as the copula (cop.). It may appear in contracted form, e.g. He's (symbolized as 'cop.').

The difference between an object and a complement can be seen from the following examples:

> *I called him a fool.*   (i.e. 'You are a fool')   *I called him a taxi.*
> S V   O   C   S V O_i O_d

(The latter does not imply 'You are a taxi'!)

There are other kinds of complementation, with different functions from the above, but they need not concern us here. The most important one is to express the agent, usually introduced by 'by', as in:

He was seen by the policeman.
S   V   C

8   A very few verbs govern an ADVERBIAL (A)—a word or phrase indicating time, manner, place, etc., as in:

He put it on the table.   *They lived in the sixteenth century.*
S V O   A   S   V   A

In all other cases, adverbials are optional elements of clause structure: they have no effect on the classification of the sentence; they may be omitted, and the sentence would still be grammatically acceptable (though of course its meaning would have slightly altered), as in:

He walked quickly.   *He walked.*
S   V   A   S   V

He soon saw the answer.   *He saw the answer.*
S A V   O   S V   O

There may of course be more than one adverbial in a clause, as in:

They walked home quickly at three o'clock.
S   V   A   A   A

9   The last element of clause structure is also optional—the VOCATIVE (Voc).

John, I asked you a question.   *Come here, Mr Jones.*
Voc S V O_i O_d V   A   Voc

10   So far, we have said little about the order in which these elements occur. The following guidelines should therefore be noted.

(*i*) S goes after the first part of any verb in *Questions*. 'The first part of a verb' here means the AUXILIARY verbs (*be, have, may, can, do,* etc.), symbolized as Aux. Example:

Is he coming?   *Can the boys get here?*
Aux S V   Aux   S   V A

S goes before the verb everywhere else, with a few minor exceptions.

(*ii*) O and C go after the verb. If they cooccur, O usually goes before C.

(*iii*) A usually occurs at the end of the sentence, but it may sometimes be found in other positions (e.g. for emphasis), as in:

Quickly John came home.   John *quickly* came home.
John came *quickly* home.

(*iv*) Voc usually goes either at the very beginning or at the very end of a sentence.

11 The basic structure of a clause may now be summarized as:

$$(Voc)^9 + SV + \begin{cases} O \\ C \\ A \end{cases} + \begin{cases} O \\ C \\ A \end{cases} + (A)^9$$

12 Multiple sentences consist of more than one clause; but each clause is of exactly the same basic pattern as that just outlined.

Multiple sentences are traditionally classified into two types:

(*i*) sentences with clauses linked by a *coordinating* device (mainly *and, or, but*), symbolized here with a small c, as in:

> *John came at three and we came later.*
> S   V   A   c   S   V   A

(*ii*) sentences where all clauses except one are *subordinate*; that is, they depend upon a 'main' clause for their occurrence, and are linked with it through a subordinating device (such as 'because', 'how'), symbolized here with a small 's'.

But before illustrating this, we must note what 'depend upon' means: it means that the clause is *part of* the structure of the main clause. In all the examples so far, the elements of clause structure (S, V, O, C, A, Voc) have always been single words or short phrases. But sometimes an element of structure can be itself a clause. This can be seen clearly from the following set of examples:

> Mary walked *quickly.*
> Mary walked *at a rapid pace.*
> Mary walked *because there was no bus.*
> S   V   A

All three sentences contain adverbials; but in the first, the adverbial is simply an adverb; in the second, it is an adverbial phrase; and in the third, it is an adverbial clause. Here is another example:

> *That*   was interesting.
> *The news*   was interesting.
> *What he said* was interesting.
> S   V   C

All three sentences contain subjects; but in the first, the subject is a single word, a pronoun; in the second, it is a noun phrase (see below); and in the third, it is a noun clause.

So in the analysis of multiple sentence structure, *two* levels of depth must be introduced into the analysis: one must say both what the structure of the main clause is, and *then* what the structure of any dependent clause is, as follows:

> *Mary ran, because she was late.*
> S   V   A
>   s   S   V   C

---

[9] Brackets indicate the optional elements of structure.

Multiple sentences may of course be built up indefinitely:

> *He came at three when he had realized the time,*
> S   V   A   ——————— A ———————
>   s   S   V   O

> *and John asked him what he wanted.*
> c   S   V O_i ——— O_d———
>   s   S   V

There may even be dependent clauses within dependent clauses, as in:

> *He laughed when he heard that the book was finished.*
> S   V   ———— —   A ————————————
>   s   S   V   O
>   s   S   V

It should be noted that dependent clauses can replace any of the elements of clause structure except the verb:

replacing S: *That we need food is obvious. What I said was . . .*
replacing O: *We saw that she was happy. Let us know where you live.*
replacing C: *The point is that we're leaving.* (The 'that' may be omitted.) *I found him reading the paper.*
replacing A: *When we return, I'll tell you.*

They may also occur *with* an element of clause structure, e.g. as a relative clause (e.g. The men *who came*) or appositional (e.g. the question, *whether we need it, . . .*).

Not all dependent clauses are of the type illustrated so far (the so-called 'finite clauses'). The following deserve separate mention.

(*i*) a 'non-finite clause'—that is, one introduced by a participle or an infinitive form of the verb, as in:

> *Walking down the road, I saw John. To err is human.*
> ————   A   S V O   S V C
> V   A   V

When this is in object position, there are many possibilities, depending on the type of verb used, e.g.

> *He likes to talk. He likes talking to people. I saw her coming. I want him to go.*

(*ii*) a 'verbless clause'—that is, one where the verb is implicit, as in:

> *Although anxious, he still went.* (i.e. 'Although he was anxious . . .')
> ———— A   S A V
>   s   C

(*iii*) a 'comparative clause', which has an idiosyncratic pattern of clause linkage, as follows:

> *This is bigger than that is.*
> S   V   C

Cf. also *He is less happy than he was. He was as pleased as she was. It goes so fast that . . . This is more interesting than that,* all of which we analyse as SVC. Note, however, the following structure, where we analyse the clause as A:

> *So many people came that we closed the door.*
> S   V   A

(*iv*) 'comment clauses', e.g. *you know, mind you, to be fair, as you say*; their parenthetic status suggests the following transcription:

> *He came at six, you see.*
> S   V   A   (S V)

(*v*) clauses commencing with the 'empty' items, *it* and *there* need a separate classification, because of their idiosyncratic relationship to other sentences, e.g.

> *it's raining   there were many people there*
> it   V   there V   C   A

13   Minor sentences. These are of various kinds. They usually lack the characteristic SV pattern of the major sentence; and if they do have a SV structure, this tends to be fixed—the sentence is incapable of making the structural changes that a major sentence can normally undergo (e.g. *Bless you!* after a sneeze is not part of a pattern *I bless* etc.). Examples:

Stereotypes
(*i*) Restricted patterns, e.g. *What about* it? *Down with* him! *You and your* books!
(*ii*) Aphorisms, e.g. The more the merrier. Easy come, easy go.
(*iii*) Learned utterances, e.g. nursery rhymes.

Social
(*i*) Phrases for greeting, thanking, exclaiming etc., e.g. Goodbye. Merry Christmas. Help! Sorry. Mind! Pardon. Blast! Goal! Well, well.
(*ii*) Interjections, e.g. Tut-tut. Oh! Ugh!
(*iii*) Vocatives, e.g. John!
(*iv*) Responses: Yes. No. Mhm.

These patterns cannot be given any useful subclassification. They must simply be listed.

14   Sentence connection. There are four main ways of connecting sentences together.

(*i*) Using pronunciation, by linking them with intonation, e.g.

> John said he'd cóme.   Mary said she'd stày.

(In writing, we may use space, colour etc. to link sentences.)

(*ii*)   Using vocabulary, replacing a word in one sentence by a related word in the next, as in:

> *Georgie Best* is still abroad.   *The handsome footballer* has not been . . .

(*iii*)   Using commonsense semantic connection, as in:

> He died on Thursday.   He was buried on Saturday.

(The reverse order would be rather unlikely.)

(*iv*)   Using grammatical links, of which there are three main kinds:

> (*a*)   Adverbials of time, place, consequence etc.
>
> > John came in.   *Then* Bill went out.
>
> (*b*)   Cross-reference, using articles, pronouns etc.
>
> > John came in.   *He* was angry.
> > I saw a cat in the road.   *The* cat was angry.
> > I want a book.   Can you get me *one*.
> > John drives a car.   I *do* too.

(*c*)   A major sentence may omit elements of clause structure when these are present in a previous sentence. This ability to leave bits out of a sentence (referred to as *ellipsis*) is very important.

> *Where   are   you going?   To town.*   (i.e. I'm going to town)
> Q   S   V   A
>
> *Who's in the bathroom?   John.*   (i.e. John is in the bathroom)
> Q V   A   S

Elliptical major sentences are usually responses which aim to avoid repetition of a previous sentence. They should not be confused with minor sentences, which are not derivable from a previous major sentence: in elliptical sentences, the elided words are uniquely recoverable, or the context allows a very small set of alternatives, e.g. *Lunch?* (i.e. 'Are you ready for lunch', etc.)

15   Phrase structure. We must now ask: what may occur as an element of clause structure?
What may be a Subject?

(*i*)   One or more pronouns, e.g. *He/This/Someone* is coming.
(*ii*)   One or more noun phrases. A noun phrase (NP) consists of a noun along with any words which are dependent upon it, e.g. adjectives, articles (see further below): *The boy* is coming. *John* is ready.
(*iii*)   One or more dependent clauses, e.g. *What I said* was obvious. *To walk* was impossible.
(*iv*)   An 'empty' item, *it* or *there*, e.g. *it*'s raining, *there* were twenty.

Certain of these may be combined, e.g. *The boy and I* . . . Coordination may be explicit (using a conjunction) or implicit, as with 'apposition', e.g. *John, the butcher,* is over there (see *GCE* 9.130ff., *UGE*, 9.45ff.).

What may be an Object?

(*i*)   All the patterns that occur as subject apart from (*iv*), but

(*ii*)   Some of the pronouns change their form, e.g. *He* asked *him*.

(*iii*)   The direct–indirect object construction (note that indirect objects may only be NPs or pronouns).

What may be a complement?

(*i*)   The same as in object patterns (*i*) and (*ii*), with a few other structures possible, e.g. adjective constructions (e.g. *He is happy*), the comparative clause.

(*ii*)   A *prepositional phrase*, i.e. a noun-phrase preceded by a preposition:

He was seen *by the man*

What may be an adverbial?

An adverb, adverbial phrase (which may be either NP or preposition + NP) or adverbial clause, as illustrated above.

What may be a verb?

Only a verb phrase, i.e. a main verb, with any accompanying auxiliary verbs and negative particles. Auxiliaries are symbolized by Aux; negatives by Neg. The main verb has a small v, to distinguish it from the capital V, which stands for the whole element of clause structure.

He might not have been coming.
S _____ __ ____ _____
V
Aux Neg Aux Aux   v

16   The two main bits of structure to be analysed further are the Noun Phrase (NP) and the Verb Phrase (VP). Note how important NP may be in a sentence:

The man   gave   the boy   a book   in the morning.
NP (as S)   NP (as O_i) NP (as O_d)   NP (as A)

17   **Structure of the Noun Phrase.** There are three main positions: the centre or 'head' which is the noun; the dependent words which precede it ('premodification'); and the dependent words which follow it ('postmodification.). Examples:

Premodification	*Head*	*Postmodification*	
	Buns		taste nice.
The	buns	in the window	taste nice.
All those lovely currant	buns	in the window of the shop	taste nice.

It is clear that NPs can get indefinitely large, and require further analysis.

18   **Nouns.** These are described with reference to four main kinds of contrast:

(*i*)   *Number*: singular–plural, e.g. *boy–boys, man–men* (transcription symbol: pl.);

(*ii*)   *Case*:   whether possession is marked, e.g. *boy/boy's/boys'* (transcription symbol: gen., for 'genitive');

(iii)   Gender: whether the noun patterns with *he/she/it* (e.g. *boy–he, girl–she, boat–it/she*);

(iv)   Type: whether the noun is proper/common, concrete/abstract, mass/count (e.g. *wheat/oats*) etc.

These categories will not be analysed further in the present approach: they are fully illustrated in *GCE/UGE* in the following sections: *(i)* 4.48ff./4.31ff. *(ii)* 4.93ff./4.66ff.   *(iii)* 4.85ff./4.58ff.   *(iv)* 4.2ff., 4.28ff./4.16ff.

An adjective may also function as head of a NP, e.g. *The fastest* gets the prize.

Personal pronouns function to replace NPs as wholes (not just single nouns) and are rarely modified. Note however the phenomenon of 'reflexive' modification, using *reflexive pronouns*, which may occur as S, O or C, e.g.

> *He shaved himself.   He allowed himself no rest.   He is always himself.*
> $\quad$ S $\quad$ V $\quad\quad$ O$_d$ $\quad\quad$ S $\quad$ V $\quad\quad$ O$_i$ $\quad\quad$ O$_d$ $\quad\quad$ S V A $\quad\quad$ C
>
> *He himself couldn't come.*
> $\quad$ S $\quad\quad\quad$ V

Various other categories of pronoun are sometimes distinguished (see *GCE* 4.106ff., *UGE* 4.78ff.):

(a)   possessive (e.g. *my, your*) and *demonstrative* (e.g. *this*) when used within the NP we include under our category of Determiner below. (When used without the rest of the NP, e.g.

> *This* is interesting.   It's *mine.*
> $\,$ S $\,$ V $\quad$ C $\quad\quad$ S V $\,$ C

they are classified as Pronouns.)

(b)   relative pronouns introduce relative clauses, included under Postmodification below (these are transcribed as s, in the same way as any other dependent clause markers).

(c)   indefinite pronouns constitute a rather miscellaneous category, e.g. *everything each, much, many, few, several, enough, somebody, one* (e.g. I want one of them), *some/any, nobody, none.* They may function in the NP as Initiators or Determiners (see below). In isolation they are classified as Pronouns functioning as S, C or O, e.g.

> *We have enough.   Few know.*
> $\,$ S $\quad$ V $\quad\quad$ O $\quad\quad$ S $\quad$ V

As heads of NPs, they may be modified, e.g.

> *Someone I know is . . .*
> $\quad\quad\quad\quad$ S $\quad\quad$ V
> $\overline{\text{Pron} \quad \text{S V}}$

(d)   interrogative pronouns, e.g. *who*'s coming, we class under the general heading of Question-words, labelled as Q above.

19   Premodification. There are three main positions within this category.

Initiators (I)	*Determiners* (D)	*Adjectivals* (Adj)

e.g. all, half, double, three-fifths (± of); includes 'restrictives', e.g. only, and some intensifiers, e.g. quite, such, what, as in *what a storm*!	e.g. this/that/these/ those/a/the/no/my/ your/every/each/either/ much/what/enough . . .	Ordinals:
		  first . . . , (an)other, next, last.
		Quantifiers:
		  one, two . . . , many, few, little, several.
		Adjectives:
		  old, big, happy. . . .
		Nouns (or other word classes modifying the Head Noun (and labelled NN in transcription):
		garden shed, *railway* station, the *club* president.
		Nouns expressing possession (also labelled NN):
		vicar's hat.

Note the different classification of some items, depending on position in the sentence, e.g.

> *Enough bread.*   *Enough of the bread.*   We have *enough.*
>   D   N   I   D   N   Pron

> *Many people.*   *Many of the people.*   *The many people.*   *Many came.*
>   D   N   I   D   N   D Adj N   Pron

Some examples in full:

> *The big boys came.*   *All of the man's pockets were . . .*
>   S   V   S   V
> D Adj N   I   D Adj   N

> *Not quite all of the fat man's three big pockets were . . .*
>   S   V
>   I   D   Adj Adj Adj   N

Note that here, some of the positions require further subclassification, e.g. in the last example *fat man's* is itself a noun phrase, functioning as an adjectival—
>   Adj N

a process which could be extended indefinitely, as in 'my fat uncle's small daughter's little train . . .'.

A fairly common point not mentioned so far is that words which are dependent on adjectives are in this approach called Intensifiers (Int), e.g. The *very* big man..., The *awfully* pretty girl . . . They may also premodify other words, e.g. adverbs (*very* nicely), prepositions (*right* through).

20   Postmodification. There are two main structures:

(*i*)   a prepositional phrase, e.g.

> the man *in the garden*, the hands *of the man*;
> D N Pr D   N   D   N Pr D N

note the use of 'complex' prepositions, e.g. *in spite of* (see *GCE* 6.5ff., *UGE* 6.4).

Pr

(*ii*)   a dependent clause: finite, e.g.

the boys who saw us ran away.

S   V   A

s   V   O

non-finite, e.g.

the boys walking down the road saw a dog.

S   V   O

V   A

D   N   v   Pr   D   N

verbless, e.g.

the boys, ready for trouble, arrived.

S   V

C

D   N   Adj   Pr   N

(Note that some adjectives may also postmodify, as in: anyone *intelligent*, the men *present*; also some adverbs, especially of measure, e.g. a week *ago*, someone *else*, the way *back*.)

21   **Structure of the Verb Phrase.** Only Premodification operates in the VP. It involves expressing the following range of contrasts:

(*i*)   Tense: past tense forms (e.g. I *walked/took*) are symbolized as *-ed*; past particle forms (e.g. *walked* in *I have walked, taken* in *I have taken*) are symbolized as *-en* (see *GCE* 3.23ff., *UGE* 3.26ff.); the *have/had* here are included under the general heading of *Aux*.

(*ii*)   Aspect: a form of *be* + present participle form of the main verb, e.g. he is going (*GCE* 3.36ff., *UGE* 3.26ff.); the transcription marks *Aux* for the forms of *be*, and *-ing* to show the word structure of the participle.

(*iii*)   Mood: one of the 'modal' auxiliary verbs—*may, might, can, could, shall, will, dare, ought, need* . . . (*GCE* 3.43ff., *UGE* 3.48ff.); all are subsumed under *Aux*.

(*iv*)   Voice: active vs. passive, the latter using a form of *be* + past participle, e.g. *he is kicked* (*GCE* 2.24ff., *UGE* 7.5).

(*v*)   Negation: usually *not*, sometimes contracted to *n't* (*GCE* 2.21ff., *UGE* 2.20); symbolized as *Neg/n't* respectively.

(*vi*)   Number: third person singular (symbolized as *3s*) v. other persons, e.g. *goes, walks*.

(*vii*)   Other, more complex constructions (e.g. *he might have to be asked*)

Aux   Aux   Aux   v

which are not analysed further here, each item being marked with Aux; no separate transcription is given to the marker *to*.

Note that the main verb may have more than one word, being followed by a 'particle' (part), as in *come down* (='descend'), *get up to* (*What does he get up to*)

v   part   v part part

etc. It is important to distinguish multiword verbs which end in a preposition from verbs followed by a prepositional phrase, e.g.

> *He looked over the room* (='examined')
> S   V   O
>   v   part D N

> *He looked over the river* (='gazed across').
> S   V   A
>   Pr D N

The distinction is sometimes ambiguous, e.g. *He came across the road* (='on foot'? 'on a map'?). Note also that *part* is often separated from the lexical verb, e.g.

> *He looked me over*
> S   V   O
>   v   part

A full classification of irregular verbs is in *GCE* 3.63ff., *UGE* 3.10ff.

(Note also that *Aux* forms may be contracted, e.g. *he's coming, he'll go*; these are symbolized as *'aux*.)

22   Word structure. The main point to note is the use of the following:

In the NP: Plural (pl), Genitive (gen), Comparative (-er)–Superlative (-est) (e.g. *bigger–biggest*).

In the VP: third person present singular (3s), present participle form (-ing), past participle form (-en), past tense (-ed), and contracted forms of the auxiliary ('aux), copula ('cop) and negative (n't).

The objective (or 'accusative') case in some pronouns, e.g. *he–him*.

The adverb marker -ly, e.g. *beautifully*.

D Major sentence function

We recognize four main functions for major sentences:

(*i*)   *statements*, using the various simple and multiple types already illustrated.

(*ii*)   *questions* (see *GCE* 7.53ff., *UGE* 7.43ff.). There are four main ways of forming a question:

> (*a*)   SV becomes Aux + S + V, e.g. *He's coming—Is he coming?* This is symbolized as SV at clause level, the auxiliary placement appearing in the analysis at phrase level, as follows:

Is he coming?

<u>S</u> <u>V</u>
Aux Pron v

(*b*) Using a question-word (Q, e.g. *what, how, when, why*) along with SV inversion, as in:

He's coming.   When is   he   coming?
S   V   Q   <u>S</u>   <u>V</u>
                   Aux Pron   v

(*c*) Using intonation—usually a rising tone instead of a falling one (best symbolized by an accent over the element carrying the question-tone), as in: *He's còming. He's cóming?* It should be emphasized, however, that this use of intonation is not a matter of syntax, but of attitude—in this case, a 'questioning' or 'puzzled' attitude—signalled by the rising tone. That the use of a rising tone on a statement does not amount necessarily to a question is clearly shown by the use of the same tone to indicate, for example, shocked surprise or excited emphasis (see further, Crystal 1969, ch. 8). Only the context can resolve which attitude is involved.

(*d*) Tag-questions, along with rising intonation, e.g. *isn't he, aren't they?*

He's coming, ísn't he?
S   V   V   S

(*iii*) *commands* (see *GCE* 7.72ff., *UGE* 7.58ff.). There are four types:

(*a*) With no subject, as already illustrated, e.g. *Go!*

(*b*) With an indefinite subject, e.g. *Someone shut the door!*

S V_{imp} O

(Note that we need to transcribe V_{imp} here, to distinguish it from SVO as such, which would look like an ordinary statement.)

(*c*) With verb *let*, as in: *Let's go!* Here, as in the case of *do* below, we have

let   V

a unique usage in English; we therefore transcribe it fully, rather than calling it an Auxiliary, which would be misleading.

(*d*) With verb *do*, as in: *Do come in!*

do   V

(*iv*) *exclamations* (see *GCE* 7.78, *UGE* 7.63). There are only two exclamatory sentences of the major type (NB: exclamatory words, noises etc. are classed under Minor sentences above). These are introduced by *What* and *How*, as in:

What a nice place this is!   How nicely she jumps!
Q   C   S   V   Q   A   S   V

In Appendix D (p. 207), we give a sample of adult dialogue analysed in the above terms. Each sentence is analysed at the three main levels of sentence/clause, phrase and word, and the transcription to be made at each level is indicated vertically.

The prosodic analysis

Because of the importance of intonation in assessing the nature of a disorder as well as the degree of successful interaction between T and P (see below), it is essential that all speech data is given a transcription of the major prosodic features. We do not want too detailed or 'narrow' a transcription: there is simply no time to do routine prosodic analysis of a very detailed sort, and in any case we are not sure that there would be any point, as we have so far found only the grosser prosodic features to be of clinical relevance. We therefore give systematic recognition only to a subset of prosodic features—to intonation, rhythm and pause, in particular. Other features (such as speed, voice quality) which may from time to time be significant, we note on an ad hoc basis, using the transcription sheet margins (see chapter 5).

Under the heading of *intonation*, we mark:

(*i*)   the main melodic contours into which any stream of speech can be divided. These are called tone-units, and their boundaries are marked in our transcription by /. They are often followed by a pause. Example:

John came at three/ Mary came at four/ and Albert at five/

(*ii*)   Within each tone-unit, one word (occasionally two) is spoken with greater prominence than all the others, and we mark this *nucleus* by placing on it the *nuclear tone*, which indicates the general direction of pitch at this point. This tone may be of many kinds, but we regularly indicate only *falling*, *rising*, *level*, and *falling-rising* pitch movements, as these are the ones which are most frequent and most functional in the expression of grammatical relationships. The above example, with one possible set of tones marked,[10] would be:

John came at thrée/ Mary came at fóur/ and Albert at five/

(*iii*)   The remaining words in the tone-unit are marked with ' if they are stressed; their pitch levels are not further shown:

'John 'came at thrée/ 'Mary 'came at fóur/ and 'Albert at five/

(*iv*)   Major distinctions in pause are marked: . is used if the pause is brief, — if it is relatively long equivalent to a pulse of the speaker's rhythm), and — —, — — — etc. for proportionately longer pauses.

These distinctions are explained in greater detail elsewhere (e.g. Crystal 1969, Crystal and Davy 1975, where there is a tape recording available). We recognize that it takes some practice before one can notate the prosodic features of speech rapidly and consistently, but we strongly recommend that T should increase his awareness of the role of these features in speech as much as possible. Trying to do without them leads to transcriptions of data that are ambiguous and that omit significant information. The only alternatives are, after all, to use ordinary punctuation, or to use no punctuation at all. The latter hardly commends itself;

---

[10] The tone is marked over the vowel of the stressed syllable.

but the former is very misleading. We have already seen (p. 43) how punctuation makes decisions which may not be present in speech; for example, is an utterance one sentence or two? And with the more loosely organized kinds of discourse, the limitations of normal punctuation show up very readily. In reading papers on adult aphasic speech, for instance, we have been at a loss to interpret such marks as . . . , which are often used to symbolize the disjointedness of P's discourse. It is not possible to understand how far P is systematically and confidently understanding T's utterance or imposing a structure on his own output without taking intonation into account. Nor can one expect to be in full control over the verbal behaviour of P if T is unaware of his own intonation and rhythm. For example, presenting a stimulus sentence for imitation requires that the original prosody be adhered to in any repetition by T. To a child at the very early stages of language awareness, what to an adult might seem a casual and unimportant modulation of rhythm or pitch can fundamentally alter the identity of the sentence. For instance, the sentences 'put the grèen 'brick 'down/ and 'put the 'green 'brick dòwn/ may, despite the similarity, sound worlds apart to a child attuned only to gross differences in phonetic form, viz. '\"' vs. '\"'.[11]

Apart from the prosody, we have not found it necessary to use phonetic transcription as a routine, as our analysis can be made independently of any segmental phonetic considerations, for the most part. However, in cases where the utterance is uncertain or incomplete, we do use a phonetic transcription, to avoid too much reading in; we also do this wherever a phonetic feature of potential grammatical significance is used variably by the speaker, e.g. if his articulation of final -s vacillates (in view of the importance of this feature for the construction of plurals, possessives etc. in English). Under these circumstances, we use a broad phonetic transcription, based on Gimson 1970.

[11] That disordered patients, child and adult, do react in such ways, is well attested. We have our own examples below, but in addition one might cite Goodglass et al. (1967), who showed that the prosodic characteristics of function words determined whether they were lost or retained in agrammatic speech; Stark et al. (1967), who showed that in cases of sequencing difficulty due to P forgetting the first item in a sequence, recall was improved when this item was given prosodic prominence. See also Blasdell and Jensen (1970).

4

The development of syntax in children

Bibliographies of child language studies show very clearly that research into the development of syntax is for the most part concentrated in the mid-1960s and subsequently. A convenient retrospect of much of this work, on early development, is to be found in Brown 1973, and other reviews are available in Dale 1972, Menyuk 1971 and Ferguson and Slobin 1973. Brown in particular paints a very clear picture of the strengths and weaknesses of this research. It is evident that there are still major gaps in our knowledge of the acquisition of certain syntactic structures and categories, but the general outline of syntactic development is fairly firmly established, and there is sufficient detail accumulated, in our opinion, to warrant investigations such as our own.

One theoretical conclusion has been particularly important for us. It is now generally held that the order of acquisition of the syntactic patterns of a language is 'approximately invariant' (Brown 1973, 58). This claim is based on a great deal of evidence for English; how far it is a general claim for all languages remains to be seen. The operative word here is 'order'. We have already had cause to point to the differences which exist in terms of *rate* of acquisition. The suggestion is that all normal children, regardless of how quickly or slowly they are travelling, are following a single developmental path.[1] Some may pass over a stage quickly; some may spend a great deal of time at a particular point; some may miss out stages altogether; some may temporarily rush ahead of themselves and use a few patterns from a later stage of development before continuing at their normal rate; some may go back a stage, for a short while; different strategies may be used in order to arrive at a given stage; and so on. But the general progression is stable. Syntactic development was once (imaginatively!) likened to a family stroll through a park; at any given point the children may be in various positions beside, behind, or in front of the parents, but the same general direction is being maintained, and ultimately the same distance will have been covered. The evidence for this view we find convincing, but we should make it clear that only the first five years of life have been studied in sufficient detail to warrant this conviction. There is every suggestion that subsequent syntactic development until puberty is also governed

[1] This is not the place to launch into a discussion about the theoretical definition of normalcy. Our statement should be interpreted operationally: by 'normal' we mean children whose language development, in the context of their home background, has given no cause for concern, and whose general psychological and physical development has been considered to fall within normal limits (as defined by the standards appropriate to those areas). See further ch. 5.

by some underlying set of conditions, but evidence on this point has yet to be accumulated. Our procedure, then, will be able to offer its more precise suggestions for the earlier stages of syntactic development, where more of the facts are known. As the disordered child's syntax approaches the 5-year-old stage, there will come a point when our approach reduces to little more than a series of informed guesses. This does not bother us unduly. There is plenty to be done to get P up to the equivalent of a 5-year-old, and as the really serious problems are located in the middle stages of syntactic development, we are happy to concentrate our attention here, and leave refinement of the later stages until more empirical findings have come in.

Our approach, then, is a descriptive synthesis of what has been discovered about the order and rate of syntactic development. Here we would draw attention to the implications of the word 'descriptive'. It is opposed here to 'theoretical'. We have not found it helpful in our work to look for theoretical explanations of language acquisition. We are aware that the child-language literature has for some years been concerned to weigh the merits and demerits of the various accounts of why language is acquired in the way it is. In particular, there has been the controversy between the behaviourist accounts of acquisition and the view that the process is essentially innate, a controversy which began with Chomsky's review of Skinner (see Chomsky 1957b; for a more recent summary, Chomsky 1968) and which still continues (see the critique in Derwing 1973). More recently, a third view, which sees language development as based on the prior development of a set of cognitive principles and strategies, and associated especially with Piaget, has been developed (see Sinclair-de-Zwart 1969). The point we want to make is that it is possible to carry out descriptions of the various features of syntactic development without having to commit oneself to any one of these theories, or any other. Whether we feel that the facts of syntax are best explained by postulating some prestructuring of the brain towards language, present at birth, or not, is a separate question from the empirical task of establishing these facts in terms of some framework of syntactic description. The theoretical questions are fascinating, but they are of little practical value when it comes to assessing a language disorder.[2] Presumably this is because none of the theories has been worked out in sufficient detail for the relationship between general explanation and empirical findings to be apparent. If and when specific hypotheses are developed and tested to indicate the nature of this relationship, we might find ourselves much helped by the postulates of these theories; but at the moment we find the theoretical discussion continuing at too abstract a level to be directly applicable to remedial problems.

[2] They are of greater practical importance when it comes to working out techniques of remediation; but here we have found eclecticism to be most beneficial. Developing cognitive strategies, using transformational drills, and presenting imitation tasks for rewards are not, in the remedial situation, mutually exclusive.

In a different theoretical connection, when we describe the increase in the number of elements of syntactic structure between stages, we do not feel it necessary to commit ourselves to whether the controlling factors are due to memory, perception, linguistic complexity etc. (see further below).

The aim of the exercise, then, is to hypothesize a set of syntactic stages through which children pass in their progress towards the adult language, and to classify the structures and categories which operate at each stage, thus providing a *syntactic profile chart* of development. But first we should make it clear that we are using the notion of 'stages' very much as a descriptive convenience. The stages are not to be viewed as discrete entities, periods of ability which switch off and on, like a sequence of relays. Syntactic development is a continuous process, and our stages are arbitrary divisions along it. The validity of these divisions can be argued on two counts. Firstly, there is a theoretical justification, that each stage corresponds to some general linguistic process which it is possible to identify in formal terms. Secondly, there is pragmatic justification: using these stages provides a workable scheme for assessment and remediation. The theoretical point is also the one made by Brown (1973, 59), though his stages are by no means identical with ours: 'A stage is. named . . . either for a process that is the major new development occurring in that interval or for an exceptionally elaborate development of a process at that stage.' A stage 'derives its name from the process that seems to dominate it' (180). In our procedure, the stages are given chronological limits, also: thus, Stage I goes from 0;9 to 1;6 ('nine months' to 'one year and six months'); Stage II from 1;6 to 2;0; and so on. It is therefore possible—and indeed expected— for the signs of development of the linguistic processes falling within a stage to be seen before the chronological onset of that stage; and of course many (not all) of the structures which have emerged within a stage will continue to be used after that stage, and throughout the adult language. The model of stages thus looks something like this:

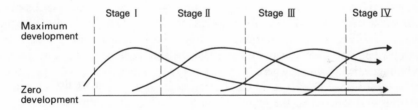

Certain Stage I and II patterns continue to be used throughout later stages; rather more State III patterns are retained; even more Stage IV patterns; and so on. The point here is the obvious one, that the later a pattern is to be acquired, the more likely it will be to approximate towards the adult language, and therefore stay without change. There is presumably some normal ratio of patterns from the various stages which characterizes samples from any one stage. For example, at Stage III there may be 10 per cent Stage I patterns, 20 per cent Stage II patterns, 60 per cent Stage III patterns, 10 per cent Stage IV patterns. From the samples we have analysed so far, and from the literature, all we can assert with any confidence is the dominant statistic for a stage: at least 60 per cent of the structural processes found in a Stage will be those belonging to that Stage. The exact ratios of the remainder have not as yet been worked out.

Seven Stages are recognized, and are described in terms of the descriptive framework outlined in chapter 3. This, however, is by no means an unproblematic decision, and we perhaps ought to clarify how we view the status of the Syntactic Profile Chart, to avoid its being attributed claims we do not intend it to make. The chart outlined below is essentially a summary of syntactic developments which have been noted in children, and the categories outlined in chapter 3 are seen as no more than a convenient means of identification of these developments. The chart is a grid on which progress in syntax can be measured; but it is not an arbitrary grid, as one might find on, say, an ordnance survey map. The points recognized on the chart are motivated by our being able to establish patterns of formal and semantic correspondence between them and analogous points in the adult language, correspondences which become increasingly clear as the child matures. At the beginning of the language-learning process, the syntactic correspondences between child and adult are naturally very approximate: the child's categories might be said to be the 'protoform' of the adult's, by which term we are trying to suggest the existence of a general semantic/structural correspondence (as evidenced by some degree of mutual intelligibility between adult and child, and consistency in the child's use of certain formal features, such as word-order), but no one-to-one equivalence between the syntactic properties of the adult system and those of the child. The child's N, S, V etc. are similar to the adult's in certain respects only (cf. McNeill's (1966) notion of a 'generic' relationship between classes), and the approximation becomes increasingly accurate over time. Deciding on the point when the child's syntactic system may be said to be sufficiently close to that of the adult to warrant a confident analysis in adult terms is by no means easy, however. We take the view that by the end of our Stage II below there is sufficient consistency in the child's use of linguistic forms, and sufficient stability in the adult's interpretation of these forms, to be satisfied that a description in terms of S, V, Pr, N etc. is not too misleading. This is in fact a fairly conservative position when one compares it with some of the claims made in the contemporary psycholinguistic literature, where there is a ready tendency to attribute a great deal of structural knowledge to early child utterances, ascribing to the child complex intentions and structures, the *linguistic* status of which it is extremely difficult to verify. It is always a tentative matter to analyse the utterances of a child in terms of a set of categories and patterns originally devised for adult language. On the other hand, it is equally unsatisfactory to wait until the child is close to adult language use before daring to use any such categories. Our position, we hope, is a reasonable compromise. We use adult terminology for the description of our Stages because there is no alternative at present available; but we do not mean to imply by this that we attribute to the child some sort of linguistic awareness of the full adult potential of the categories used. The child does not build up his language piece by piece, like a jigsaw-puzzle, with each piece fully formed. To use adult terminology inevitably gives this impression superficially; but it is an impression which can be disregarded, given the appropriate emphasis to the contrary, and it is this which is the purpose of the present paragraph.

Stage I: One-element 'sentences'

The inverted commas around the term 'sentence' reflect the controversy in the language-acquisition literature as to whether utterances containing just one element are best called 'sentences' at all. Jespersen (1922, 133), for example, provided a caustic summary of the view that they are not. 'When we say that such a word means what we should express by a whole sentence, this does not amount to saying that the child's "up" *is* a sentence, or a sentence-word. . . . We might just as well assert that clapping our hands is a sentence, because it expresses the same idea (or the same frame of mind) that is otherwise expressed by the whole sentence "This is splendid". The word *sentence* presupposes a certain grammatical structure, which is wanting in the child's utterance.' The view is also taken by Piaget (1952) for whom the single word is a personal label for a total action pattern, incapable of linguistic differentiation; and it is the basis of the argument in Bloom 1973. On the other hand, there is a considerable body of opinion that it is possible to see one-element utterances along the lines of elliptical sentences, the other elements of the sentence being left unexpressed, either presupposed in the nonlinguistic environment in which the utterance was used (as Greenfield *et al.* in press) or part of one's innate linguistic competence (as McNeill 1970). The dispute is by no means resolved, and is bound up with theoretical questions to do with the boundary-line between syntax and semantics, and the extent to which intonation patterns at this stage are sufficiently unambiguous to justify syntactic analyses.[3] We therefore leave the question open, by our use of inverted commas, but in the interests of continuity we have kept the term 'sentence' for our heading. In devising a remedial procedure, there is a great deal to be said for treating utterances containing one element as being of the same basic kind as utterances containing two or more; and strategies which make this assumption work satisfactorily enough (see chapter 6).

There are two other terminological preliminaries. Firstly, it should be noted that we do not make use of the term 'holophrase'. The 'holophrastic stage' of syntactic development is frequently referred to in the language-acquisition literature, and we find this mode of reference disconcerting: not only does it beg the theoretical question raised above (by assuming that there are 'one-word sentences', which is what holophrase means), it also emphasizes the difference between Stage I and subsequent stages instead of reinforcing the notion of continuity in the language-learning process. The move from one-element to two-element utterances (see below) is at least suggestive of a continuous process, and makes sense therapeutically; we therefore propose to recognize it terminologically by avoiding an idiosyncratic label of no subsequent value in the description of language development. Secondly, we use the term 'element' rather than 'word', as is sometimes done, partly because

[3] The whole question is reviewed by Dore (1975). The point about intonation perhaps needs an example. Here what is being referred to is the ability of the child to mean different things by *dàda* (pointing), *dādā* (with outstretched arms) and *dáda* (upon hearing a footstep outside). These meanings can be said to correspond to what will later be called statement, command and question. The difficulty is that there is no predictable correlation between these tones and the meanings given here.

of the difficulties at this stage of distinguishing clear 'word-like' units, and also again in the interests of continuity, where the important units of pattern definition later are elements of clause structure (for an apparently similar notion, see the 'critical elements index' of Foster *et al.* (n.d.). Examples of utterances (taken from various studies) which cause problems of word identification would be: *allgone* (one word or two?), *round and round* ['raũraũ],[4] *doll-doll*, *gimme* (='give me'), *ready-steady-go* [ɛ'stɛ gou] (= the name of a jumping-game). Intonationally and distributionally these all seem to be functioning as single units, even though from the point of view of adult grammar they have more than one word.

It is this concern to avoid over-analysing the child's utterances as if they were adult structures which is the main reason for the tentative nature of the analysis made of the sentences in Stage I. Our aim is to characterize the child's syntactic ability, and we therefore want to avoid attributing him too much awareness of structure before there is clear evidence that this awareness is present. For example, if a 15-month-old says *gone*, it would be unreal to say that this is the past participle of the verb *go*, and argue that the child had an awareness of the parts of the verb. But at this early stage, it might even be unreal to say that he had an awareness of verbs at all. How do we, as observers, in fact know that the child is remarking about an action? It is not uncommon for a child to make a complete misidentification (from the adult viewpoint) and use *gone* to refer to some other characteristic of the situation, e.g. calling his dish his *gone*. It is possible to be sure about syntactic knowledge either when one can ask about it (eliciting the forms of the verb, in this example) or when there is evidence in the child's own utterance patterns that the syntactic concepts are there. Evidence of the first kind, however, is not easily obtained before the age of about 3 years (but see Shipley *et al.* 1969). Evidence of the second kind would come with the emergence of contrastive patterns of word-order (e.g. *me kick daddy* v. *daddy kick me*) or in the forms of words (e.g. *boy/boys*), and such information is not reliable until well into Stage II. For these reasons, we do not use our syntactic metalanguage for the basic description of autonomous[5] single-element sentences. We do, however, indicate the ratio of adult-looking *verbs* to *nouns* and to *other word-classes* at this stage in the remedial procedure, indicating our tentativeness by putting inverted commas around the symbols 'V' and 'N'. There are two main reasons for this. One is to reflect the well-recognized distinction in psychological development between awareness of objects and awareness of changes of state, to which the noun–verb distinction will in due course primarily relate. The other is to indicate sources of potential significance for development at later stages. If there are no 'verbs' present at Stage I, for example, introducing them becomes a priority in order to get progress in

---

[4] We use a broad phonetic and not a phonemic transcription at this point to avoid making a decision about the phonemic status of the segments, which may turn out to be premature. Most of the examples in this chapter will be given in standard orthography, in fact; allowances must therefore be made, particularly during the early Stages, for immature pronunciation.

[5] 'Autonomous' is here opposed to 'elliptical'. One-element sentences at this stage of development must be distinguished from one-element sentences deriving from the ellipsis of a major sentence pattern: the classification of these is dealt with in chapter 5.

Stage II sentence structure (see further, chapter 6). Only 'nouns' and 'verbs' are felt to be sufficiently important from these points of view to warrant separate mention at Stage I: utterances which are clearly indicative of other functions than the identification of objects or change are placed together under 'Other', e.g. *there, more*; and utterances whose status in terms of these distinctions is problematic are grouped under 'Problems'.

We ought to point out, in discussing Stage I, that we have decided not to attempt to characterize this Stage in terms of the *meanings* or *functions* or *intentions* which might be attributed to the child—as is done by almost all contemporary writers on early syntactic development (see the useful summary in Brown 1973). For example, one possible classification of one-element sentences (which we experimented with ourselves for a while) was to classify them into such semantic functions as 'Identification', 'Recurrence', 'Nonexistence',[6] 'Location', 'Temporal', 'Possession' etc. There is some formal behavioural evidence, in intonation, facial expression, gesture, and so on, which might lead us in the direction of such a classification, e.g. the utterance *dada*, said while pointing to daddy's slippers, but with daddy not present in the room, plausibly suggests an interpretation of 'Possessive'. But it is not conclusive, and there are too many cases, we find, where what the child says is quite ambiguous in respect to any of the functional classifications that have been made, or where it is difficult to see how in principle one might decide between alternative interpretations, e.g. whether a child meant 'identification' or 'location' of an object. Or again, if one tries to pick a child up, and he says *No*, vigorously shaking his head and avoiding eye-contact, does this mean 'go away', 'I don't want to', 'I don't want you to', 'I'm tired', or what? The behavioural criteria are unclear, in our own observations as well as in the studies we have read, and we therefore feel it would be premature to incorporate a semantic or cognitive classification of one-element sentences into our procedure. (This might in any case be more appropriate as part of a Semantic Profile Chart, not a syntactic one.)

We must also be extremely tentative about introducing the sentential functions of statement, question and command at this stage. It is at times quite clear by the use of intonation, facial expression, gesture and general behaviour that a one-element sentence is being used with the force of a syntactic question or command. This use of intonation, gesture and so on is an important stage in general communicative development, but it is not a development in syntax as such, for reasons which have already been indicated in chapter 3 (see p. 56). It is not therefore given a separate listing on the Profile Chart, where only two functional possibilities are recognized:

(*i*) *Questions.* If the child uses a question-word on its own (usually only *where* or *what* at this period), this is counted under 'Q', the inverted commas being retained, as with other descriptive categories at this Stage.

[6] As Brown points out (1973, 170), these first three operations of reference 'have the widest possible range of application. Any thing, person, quality, or process can be named, can recur, and can disappear.' He also refers to their compatibility with the characteristics of sensori-motor intelligence (cf. Piaget 1952).

(*ii*) *Commands.* If the child uses a verb in its base form, e.g. *jump*, and the behaviour clearly indicates the interpretation of an instruction to someone/thing else, this is counted here, again with the retention of inverted commas.

(*iii*) *Minor* sentences are classified here, as they do 'not postulate any syntactic structure; the length of the minor sentence is not taken into consideration. The following three categories are counted (cf. chapter 3, p. 49).

    (*a*) *social*—greetings, responses, vocatives, e.g. *ta, yes, hello, mummy.*

    (*b*) *stereotypes*, e.g. play formulae such as *peep-bo.*

    (*c*) *problems*—classification in terms of (*a*) and (*b*) is unclear.

We have noted no cases where one-element sentences might be said to correspond in some formal way with Exclamatory sentence types (see p. 56); this column is therefore left blank for this Stage.

    We postulate chronological norms for this Stage from 0;9 to 1;6. The latter is not a cause for much dispute; it is commonly cited as a syntactic turning-point, and coincides with the end of Piagetian sensori-motor intelligence. The choice of 0;9 is to some extent arbitrary. This date reflects the point at which we feel confident that a language-specific intonational contrastivity is emerging in the production of most children. There is evidence that English, French, Chinese etc. prosodic patterns are first manifest shortly after six months (see the review in Crystal 1973a); certainly by 0;9, the vocalizations have become better defined, and repeated patterns are heard. 'Baby always makes that noise when...' and an impression of conversational ability ('What do you think he's trying to say?') are two parental impressions that emerge between six and nine months, and they are based on the awareness of specific prosodic characteristics. Identifiable 'sentence' markers, in this view, may therefore be isolated from about this time, though it may be difficult to be sure of exactly what the utterance is until a little later, due to unclear segmental articulation. 'First words' tend not to be recognized by parents until around 12 months, but a great deal of intonational and phonetic preparation has been taking place for some three months previously, and it is this we wish to reflect by placing our date for the onset of syntactic development at 0;9.

    We may summarize Stage I as follows:

Sentence Type								
Minor					*Social*	*Stereotypes*	*Problems*	
Major				Sentence Structure				
	Excl.	*Comm.*	*Quest.*	Statement				
		'V'	'Q'	'V'	'N'	Other	Problems	

The reason for this particular layout and abbreviation will be clear from chapter 5.

Stage II: Two-element sentences

Again we avoid the use of a distinguishing label for this Stage that contrasts it too sharply with the patterns of adjacent stages—we do not, in other words, wish to talk about 'telegraphic' or 'telegrammatic' speech, which gives but a partial and misleading impression of the characteristics of this Stage. The following points need to be noted, by way of commentary.

(*a*)   All patterns at this stage contain two elements of structure. Given a possible SVOA-type sentence, e.g. *daddy will kick the ball into the car*, typical sentences emerge as having any two out of the maximum four elements, viz, *daddy kick*, *daddy ball*, *daddy car*, *kick ball*, *kick car*, or *ball car*. Some are of course more probable than others, and sometimes there will be some grammatical modification of elements, e.g. *kick* [ə] *ball*, where the ə may be an article, or *ball* [ŋ] *car*, where [ŋ] may be *in*. The two elements chosen, however, will both be stressed (whereas [ə] etc. will not be), whatever order they appear in, and there will be a definable prosodic contour over the sentence, avoiding the impression of a loose unconnected sequence of lexical items.[7]

(*b*)   At Stage II, it is possible to discern the development of a hierarchy of levels of sentence structure, in that some sentences can be described solely in terms of clause-level relationships, others in terms of phrase level. Compare the two sentences:

(*1*)   *shoes there* (= the shoes are there)
(*2*)   *big shoes* (= those are big shoes).

Accepting these interpretations, for the sake of illustration, we would analyse (*1*) as SA, (*2*) as Adj N functioning as C. Diagrammatically, this is:

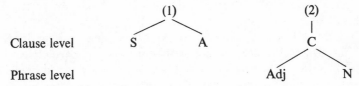

The evidence for the psychological reality of two levels of structure at this stage has been reviewed, e.g. by McNeill (1966), and is largely distributional—for instance, if the whole of the noun phrase *big shoes* were referred to by the pronoun *them*, this would suggest that the child is operating in terms of two levels of syntactic organization. Such substitutions and cross-references begin to appear in Stage II (though the main development of pronouns in fact does not take place until Stage III).

(*c*)   Given the utterance *daddy run*, where there is no doubt in a given instance

---

[7] Towards the end of Stage I, lexical items begin to string together in just such a loose way. A crucial piece of evidence for a stable grammatical relation between two lexical items is when (*a*) dominant word-order patterns emerge referring consistently to fixed sequences of situational events, and (*b*) a unifying intonation is given to the utterance (see further, Bloom 1970, 1973).

about the general meaning intended (i.e. daddy is to do the running), the question arises as to whether the child is using this sentence as an instance of the two elements Subject + Verb, or whether he is simply putting two items together, *daddy + run*. It may well be that, in the changeover from Stage I to Stage II, children pass through a period of two-word collocations, learned as wholes, e.g. *daddy run* and *pussy bite* being used before the patterns are generalized, and we get *daddy bite*, *pussy run*, etc. (see Clark *et al.* 1974). But we feel that vocabulary has increased to a sufficient size by the middle of Stage II to make very plausible the view that some productive grammatical rules have been learned (cf. McNeill 1966). We therefore are ready to talk about SV, VO etc. at this Stage, despite the possibility that at or around 1;6 some of the patterns we analyse as SV etc. may still be in the formative stage. Once again, we emphasize the tentative nature of syntactic analysis at this Stage. It will occasionally be the case that the interpretation of a two-element utterance will be syntactically unclear, e.g. whether *mummy car* is SA or NN (i.e. possessive). Intonation may help to distinguish such pairs, but not always. We do not however feel that these cases are sufficiently frequent to warrant our dispensing with syntactic analysis of this Stage altogether.

(*d*)   The notion of two-elements (and three, four below) is not a matter solely of physical length. The elements are abstract units, and the measure is thus more to do with cognitive linguistic complexity than anything else. It will usually be the case that a three-element structure will be longer in some physical sense than a two-element, e.g. in terms of morphs, or syllables, but this is not necessarily so, e.g. *'me 'go 'there* (Stage III, three syllables) vs. *daddy running* (Stage II, four syllables). There will however always be an increase in the number of stressed syllables as one moves from Stage I to Stage IV. This emphasis on element complexity is supported by Ingram (1972b), and Morehead and Johnson (1972, 153), 'The emphasis should be directed to the number of relations marked in the utterance as well as to the number of words used.'

We may now summarize the patterns we have found at Stage II. Examples here, and throughout this chapter, are partly our own, and partly taken from the acquisition literature. The general sense of an example is given in brackets when its interpretation, without situational information, would be obscure.

A   Sentence structure

1   Statement patterns

   S V, e.g. *man gone, dada running, eat doggie* (= the dog is eating).
   S O/C, e.g. *that hot, me David, boy ball* (said after a boy kicked a ball = ? the boy somethinged the ball). Note that the analytic distinction between SO and SC is entirely in terms of the kind of verb that is understood: if the verb is one of those that take complements (e.g. *be, become, seem*), the analysis is SC; otherwise SO.[8]

---

[8] This distinction is probably arbitrary at this Stage: it is unlikely that the difference between

V O/C, e.g. *want biccy, see man, ball kick, want it, give teddy* (='give it to teddy'), *be hot* (='this is hot').

A X. X is here a convenient symbol to summarize all the other elements of clause structure, S, V, O, C, with which A may cooccur. This pattern contains two elements, one of which is A, e.g. *there shoes, teddy here, put on* (='put it on top of'), *mummy car* (='mummy is in the car').

Neg X, e.g. *not dada, not run, there no, nomore train.*

Other. There are inevitably structures whose analysis, for whatever reason, is uncertain or ambiguous, and they are grouped together, along with any infrequent two-element combinations that may occur, under the 'residue' *iron* (unclear whether this meant 'that's mummy's iron' or 'mummy's ironing'). Vocative + X is a possible two-element combination, e.g. *goway man* (='go away, man'), *gimme Su-su* (='give it to me Susan'), but it is uncommon in the type of sample used in our procedure (see ch. 5).

2   *Question patterns*

Q X, e.g. *what that, where dada, pussy where.* (See Bellugi 1965, Limber 1973.)

3   *Command patterns*

V X, e.g. *jump down, kick Bonzo.*

B   Phrase structure

As with Sentence Structure patterns, each element carries a main stress.

NP[9]   N N, e.g. *mummy bag* (='mummy's bag').

Adj N, e.g. *red shoes,*[10] *big kiss.*

D N, e.g. *my ball, that man.*

VP   V V, e.g. *make run* (='make something run'), *want see* (='I want to see').

V part, e.g. *come out.*

Pr N, e.g. *in box, on table* (*in* and *on* seem to be the first two prepositions acquired by most children, cf. Brown 1973).

Int *X*, e.g. *down there, very sore.*

Other, e.g *nice big* (Adj Adj).

O and C could be clearly motivated by evidence from the child's language, as the complement-taking verbs are generally absent. Alternative analyses, e.g. by defining a new category to subsume both O and C, raise problems of their own, however. We retain the distinction, but we use it with caution.

[9] We have not attempted to subclassify Noun Phrases at this Stage in terms of whether they expound S, O, C or A. There is some evidence that more complex NPs tend to be used first in postverbal positions, and not as Subjects (cf. Limber 1973), but the picture is not entirely clear, so we have omitted this for the present.

[10] Cf. *shoes rèd*, which would suggest the analysis S C (= 'the shoes are red'). These contrasts are often difficult to be sure about, as there is unlikely to be a clear distinction in the situation, and intonation is not always unambiguous.

We may summarize Stage II as follows:

Comm.	Quest.	Statement				
V X	Q X	SV	V C/O	DN	VV	
		S C/O	A X	Adj N	V part	
		Neg X	Other	NN	Int X	
				PrN	Other	

Chronological norms for two-element sentences are postulated as being from 1;6 to 2;0.

Stage III: Three-element sentences

Two distinct processes of sentence formation account for the production of three-element sentences. One process is the blending of the patterns of Clause and Phrase Structure, which were separate from each other at Stage II; the other is the development of new patterns of Clause Structure.

A   Blends. Under this heading, we find examples such as the following:

Stage II   *see   shoes*   *red   shoes*
            V   O   O
                                       Adj N

Stage III   *see   red   shoes*
            V   O
                    Adj N

Whereas at Stage II, all elements of clause structure had been expounded by single elements at phrase structure, now an element of clause structure may be expounded by *two* elements of phrase structure. The following types of expansion are possible:

(*a*)   S expansion, e.g. *red shoes pretty* (='the red shoes are pretty').

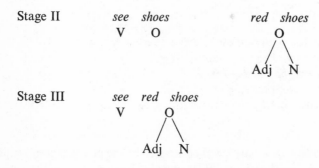

(*b*)   C/O expansion, e.g. *see that teddy*,   *Bonzo nice meat*   (='give Bonzo some nice meat')

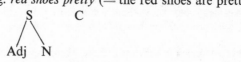

(c)   A expansion, e.g. *gone down there,   sit on chair.*

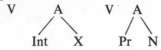

(d)   V expansion, e.g. *let man go,   why is running*

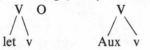

There are many possibilities of cooccurrence between the two elements of the expanded phrase and the other element of clause structure. These are not sub-classified in our approach, the label X being used to subsume the possibilities. Thus, X + S:NP is a formula which should read: 'A sentence contains two elements of clause structure: one is a Subject expounded by a two-element Noun Phrase; the other is either V, C, O, or A.' We can then summarize the above as follows:

X + S: NP
X + C/O: NP
X + V: VP
X + A: AP (Adverbial Phrase)

B   New structures: clause level. Here, three elements of clause structure are being used in sequence. Word order patterns are now fairly stable.

1   Statement patterns

S V C/O, e.g. *daddy kick ball, teddy want biccy, me get train.*
S V A, e.g *daddy gone work* (='daddy's gone to work'), *teddy sit chair.*
V C/O A, e.g. *put man chair* (='put the man in the chair').
V O_d O_i (or V O_i O_d), e.g. *give shoes David* (='give the shoes to David').
Neg X Y (where X and Y mean: any two elements of clause structure), e.g. *not ball go* (Neg S V), *no gone floor* (Neg V A = 'it's not gone on the floor'), *he not little* (S Neg C).
Others, e.g. *it broken wheels, more read book, ball big red.*

2   Question patterns

Q X Y (where X and Y identify any two elements of clause structure, or the two phrase elements of a blend; the same applies under 3 below), e.g. *what daddy going* (Q S V), *why go now* (Q V A), *where my mummy* (Q C).

When there is an Aux + V pattern at this Stage, the Aux does not invert with S, e.g. *where daddy is.* Inversion first appears separately from the question-word type of sentence (see Klima and Bellugi 1966). (It did not seem useful for our purposes to subclassify the various types of clause structure that may cooccur with question-words.)
V S, e.g. *be doggy gone* (='has doggy gone?')

3   *Command patterns*

V X Y, e.g. *put ball down* (V O A), *kick big ball* (V O).

Adj N

let X Y, e.g. *let me go* (*let* O V).

do X Y, e.g. *don't kick me* (*do* V O).

Note: Any additional information about the internal structure of three-element question or command sentences is incorporated along with the figures for statement phrase/word structure. For example, *what daddy doing* is QXY, with the *-ing* form listed under word structure; *where my daddy* is QXY, with the phrase structure noted under DN). Any additional information about clause structure, e.g. an imperative followed by a direct/indirect object construction, is not given separate classification, the possible structures concerned being extremely infrequent.

During Stage III we also find the gradual emergence of features of phrase structure that are unstable and, in a way, optional. We find, in particuar, grammatical words and inflections being introduced from the beginning of the Stage, even though they may not be stable and productive until towards the end of Stage III. Any of the above sentences may be heard with an article before a noun, for example, or the *to* form being used before the verb, or a preposition being expressed in the noun phrase, e.g. *daddy kick the ball* alongside *daddy kick ball*; *put the man in the chair* alongside *put man chair*. It would be premature to say that these grammatical modifications had been 'learned', in view of their infrequency, instability, and the errors in their use. And it is worth listening out for their occurrence, bearing in mind the potential value of this information in the remedial context, as the first appearance of such features as the article could be important. But we have not incorporated this variability into the Profile Chart.

C   New structures: phrase level

NP   N Adj N, e.g. *Johnny big train* (='Johnny's big train').
Adj Adj N, e.g. *big red ball, little black car.*
D Adj N, e.g. *that big doggy, my nice hat.*
Pr NP Pr D N, e.g. *in the corner*
Copula, e.g. *Bonzo is better, cat be hurt.*
Auxiliary, e.g. *train be going, they do go.*
Pronouns (usually in the object form, at this Stage), e.g. *me do it, him kick the ball.*

These last three categories seem to have developed sufficiently to warrant their being introduced into the procedure at Stage III, even though the development of their full use is by no means complete at this stage.

D   New structures: word level. Some inflections will have appeared sporadically at Stage II. It is not until Stage III that a sufficiently systematic pattern of usage builds up to warrant their inclusion. However, we lack detailed information about the normal order of development of the inflectional endings in English. The following order is based on Brown 1973 and the works referred to there; but it must be adopted with caution. All that can be said with confidence is that during Stages III and IV most of the inflections come to be introduced, and most of the correct patterns established. (See also Cazden 1968.)

(i) -ing, e.g. *he be **running**.* (-ing on the chart)
(ii) plural, e.g. *we saw the **girls**.* (pl.)
(iii) past tense, e.g. *that car **crashed**.* (-ed)
(iv) past participle, e.g. *it's **broken*** (-en)
(v) 3rd person singular, e.g. *he **wants** his dinner.* (3s)
(vi) possessive, e.g. *that be **teddy's** pencil.* (gen.)
(vii) contracted negative, e.g. *he **isn't** coming.* (n't)
(viii) contracted form of the copula, e.g. *he's happy.*[11] ('cop.)
(ix) contracted form of the auxiliary, e.g. *he's coming.* ('aux.)
(x) superlative forms, e.g. *that's the **biggest** one.* (-est)
(xi) comparative forms, e.g. *it's **bigger**.* (-er)
(xii) adverbial suffix, e.g. *go **quickly*** (-ly)

Stage III may be summarized as follows:

Comm.	Quest.	Statement					
		Clause			Phrase		
V X Y		X + S:NP	X + V:VP		X + C/O:NP	X + A:AP	-ing
	Q X Y	SVC/O	VC/OA		D Adj N	Cop	pl
let X Y	VS	SVA	VO$_d$O$_i$		Adj Adj N	Aux	-ed
		Neg *X Y*	Other		Pr DN	Pron	-en
do X Y					N Adj N	Other	3s
							gen
							n't
							'cop
							'aux
							-est
							-er
							-ly

The chronological range of this Stage is 2;0 to 2;6.

Stage IV: Sentences of four elements or more

As with Stage III, there are two main processes of obtaining an extra element of sentence structure: blending two patterns of the previous Stage, or developing new patterns of clause or phrase structure consisting of four or more independent elements.

[11] The development of copula ahead of auxiliary, and uncontractible *be* before the contracted form, is confirmed by Ingram (1972a).

A Blends. Exactly the same processes apply as above, with the following results.

S V O, e.g. *he lost his shoe* (O expansion)
S V A, e.g. *you writing on the board* (A expansion)
        big train gone now (S expansion)
V O_d O_i, e.g. *give teddy that car* (O expansion)
Q S V, e.g. *why it be jumping, where that man gone*

Similar formulae are used to p. 71 above, e.g. XY + S:*NP* means that the sentence contains three elements of clause structure, one being the Subject expounded by a two-element Noun Phrase, the others being any two of V, C, O or A.

B New structures: clause level

1 Statement patterns

S V C/O A, e.g. *daddy's kicking the ball now.*
S V O_d O_i, e.g. *you gave the ball to Sarah.*
A A X Y (where X and Y are any two non-adverbial elements) e.g. *me go in kitchen in a minute.*
Other. By this Stage, there are many possible permutations of elements for the clause, and it makes little sense to attempt to classify all of them separately, as they are each of low frequency, e.g. clauses with five or more elements (using sequences of adverbials, for instance). All other possibilities are counted together under this heading.

2 Question patterns

Q X Y Z, i.e. a question-word with any three other elements of structure, e.g. *where is daddy going, where my daddy going.* Inversion of SV is now normal within question-word sentences. By this Stage, also, most of the question-words are in use (cf. Ingram 1972d).

3 Command patterns

+ S, i.e. the Subject of the verb may now be expressed in a command, e.g. *you kick that ball.*

C New structures: phrase level [12]

NP   N Pr N, e.g. *man in the garden, the boy with red shoes.*
VP   2 Aux, e.g. *he have been crying.*
       Neg V, e.g. *he **not want** to, he **doesn't like** it, mummy **not gone** in the car.*

---

[12] It should be noted that once these phrase structures come to be used, they may expand elements of clause structure, as at earlier stages, e.g. *David saw teddy and doll-doll in the garden* (= S V O A). The various possible blends are now too numerous to be given separate classification.

The negative element is now beginning to be used within the verb phrase, and is no longer an appendage of the clause as a whole (cf. Klima and Bellugi 1966 for details of this process).

Pr NP   Pr D Adj N, e.g. *near the big house.*

Neg X (X = other elements of phrase structure than V), e.g. *not that pencil.*

c X (where X = any element of phrase structure), e.g. *and teddy* (i.e. teddy is to do something as well).

XcX, e.g. *teddy and dolly, wet and dirty.*

D   New structures: word level. See the discussion under Stage III. We may summarize the structures dominating Stage IV as follows:

Comm.	Quest.	Statement			
		Clause		Phrase	
		XY + S:NP XY + V:VP		XY + C/O:NP XY + A:AP	
+ S	QVS	SVC/OA	AAXY	N Pr NP	Neg V
	QXYZ	SVO$_4$O$_1$	Other	Pr D Adj N	Neg X
				cX	2 Aux
				XcX	Other

The chronological range of this Stage is 2;6 to 3;0. This makes an appropriate point at which to summarize. By 3 years, we may say, the child has come to use all the types of clause construction outlined in chapter 3. All the elements of structure have been acquired, and their pattern of distribution well established. Phrase structure is by no means so fully developed, but the main elements are present, and there has been some expansion, particularly in the premodification of the noun phrase, and particularly in postverbal positions (i.e. X(Y) + C/O:*NP* develops before X(Y) + S:*NP*. All the main sentence functions have been established, with the possible exception of exclamatory patterns. Regular word morphology patterns are now in use.

Stage V: Recursion

With the internal structure of clauses now complete, the next stage of syntactic development is the production of patterns of clause sequence, to produce the various types of multiple sentence structure which were referred to in chapter 3. Essentially what the child has to learn here is the set of connecting devices which can be used to interrelate clauses, and the transformational processes whereby one can be used within ('embedded within') another. Once these devices have been learned, of course, the process can continue indefinitely, longer and more complex sentences being built up as a result. It is this feature of language, to take a basic structure and use it repeatedly to produce extensive sequences, which is the primary characteristic of the *creativity* of language (see Lyons 1970). It is accordingly a stage of great significance in normal development, as at this point the range of expression available to the child is enormously increased. We label this Stage 'recursion', the term being taken from the literature on generative grammar, and referring to the formal characteristic of language to generate extended sentence patterns by the repeated application of a single rule.

The first recursive process that emerges at clause level is the use of coordinating conjunctions, especially *and* and *so*. We have already noticed the use of *and* in phrase structure at Stage IV, but its use is greatly restricted, and tends to be found only in fixed patterns. The first really productive use of *and* occurs at around age 3, to produce sequences such as *daddy went into the garden and the doggie chased him and—and he fell over and—* . . . As we have seen (p. 43), it is sometimes difficult to decide where a sentence begins and ends. The child seems to use *and* as a way of maintaining narrative flow; the conjunction is often attached to the *end* of a clause and followed by a pause—as if it were a sign to the listener not to interrupt while the next stage in the story is being thought up! Once it is used as a regular means of linking clauses, *and* turns up more frequently linking elements of clause structure and within phrases (*mummy and daddy* . . . , *nicely and quietly* . . . , *in a car and in a train* . . .). For this reason, we give it separate listing in our classification, distinct from the other coordinating conjunctions (e.g. *but*, *so*), and the subordinating conjunctions (e.g. *'cos*, *when*) which also develop at this stage. We therefore recognize four headings under connectivity in Stage V:

    and

    c (= other coordinating conjunctions)

    s (subordinating conjunctions)

    Other (including the other forms of linkage cited in chapter 3, p. 50, none of which are individually particularly common at this Stage, e.g. *what's that then*).

Examples of the main sentence types which emerge at Stage V are as follows:

      coordinating, e.g. *the car goes away and it comes to here.*
      subordinating, e.g. *she's sleeping 'cos she tired.*

In our classification, we make a distinction for convenience between the simplest form of clause connection, where two clauses only are conjoined, and all other connected sequences. The heading 1 therefore refers to sentences where the process of coordination or subordination occurs only once; 1 + refers to sentences where these processes have operated more than once. Examples of 1 + sentences would be: *the car goes away and it comes to here and now it's fallen over; daddy said he can come 'cos he's been a good boy.* In a more detailed analysis, it may prove necessary to subclassify these longer sequences; but this is generally unnecessary in remedial contexts.

Three other clausal developments emerge strongly at Stage V. One is the use of noun clauses as exponents of S, C, or O (cf. p. 48). These generally emerge in postverbal positions before preverbal ones. Secondly, comparative clauses begin to be used. Thirdly, within the noun phrase we find the emergence of relative clauses and the range of nonfinite clause types (cf. Brown 1971). Once again, it is possible to find these singly or in sequence, and we therefore need to make use of a convention as in the previous paragraph: 1 refers to a single instance of a post-modifying noun clause, 1 + to a sequence, as in *that car parked in the street and painted all red belongs to. . . .*

Recursion also affects phrases. We have already noted in Stages II–IV prepositional phrases of varying degrees of complexity within the noun phrase. Stage V now allows for sequences in prepositional phrases, as in *the man in the shop with a coat on.*

Under sentence types, the only new developments are twofold:

(*a*) Under the heading of questions, we note the development of tag questions, following hard upon the learning of patterns of inversion and negation in the verb phrase, which was a characteristic of Stage IV (cf. McGrath and Kunze 1973).

(*b*) The two main types of exclamatory pattern seem to emerge at around this time, but we have few instances, hence this placement must remain tentative.

Stage V may therefore be summarized as follows:

Excl.	*Comm.*	*Quest.*	*Statement*			
			Conn.	Clause		Phrase
			and	Coord. 1 1 +		Postmod. 1 1 + clause
how		tag	c	Subord. 1 1 +		
			s	Clause: S		Postmod. 1 + phrase
what			Other	Clause: C/O		
				Comparative		

As regards the chronology of this Stage, we hypothesize the period from 3;0 to 3;6. We find the latter age satisfactory, but the former is more doubtful. There is some suggestion in the literature that a much earlier onset to clause-level recursion is the case (e.g. Limber 1973 cites 2;6 to 3;6 for his patterns of embedding),[13] but we do not feel from our own data that these processes are sufficiently productive until at least 2;9 for most children. We retain 3;0 as our starting-point to maintain a clear progression in the sequence of our stages, but this may at some point have to be revised.

Stage VI: System completion

Taperecording a child of $3\frac{1}{2}$, one gets a distinct impression that the bulk of the language-learning process has taken place, and indeed comments to this effect

[13] It should be noted that Limber uses a different notion of multiple sentence: any sentence with more than one verb is a complex sentence for him—and this therefore includes some of the structures which we consider types of C.

have often been made (e.g. McNeill 1966, 15). Stable patterns of word order, along with a wide range of sentence structures and types, are at the root of this impression, and make the speech highly intelligible, so that one often fails to notice the many 'local' errors of syntax which remain to be sorted out, or the new ways in which syntactic processes already present come to be extended. The coherence of Stage VI is definable at a very abstract level, as it refers to the way in which children between 3;6 and 4;6 sort out these local syntactic problems and eradicate the vast majority of errors from their speech. Putting this another way, we can say that the child is doing so much *right* at 3½ that it is not economical to any longer describe solely in terms of what he *can* do; it is more practical to describe what he *cannot* do, as evidenced by his residual syntactic mistakes. Stage VI, then, to a great extent, reverses the direction of the analysis hitherto, incorporating information which is, in effect, a kind of error analysis.[14]

This is a stage about which information is difficult to come by. Certain areas have been researched; others remain completely unstudied. All we can do, then, is indicate the range of topics with which any procedure would have to deal at this point. The most satisfactory organization that can be imposed on the data is to talk in terms of *systems* of syntactic features, some of which the child has already begun to master, others of which he has yet to develop. This list is not complete: it incorporates only those areas of syntax which we have noted as being particularly in evidence during this period. Moreover, because we are dealing for the most part with sets of syntactic contrasts, and not just with single patterns, a checklist of occurrences or errors, as has been done in the case of Stages I–V, is of only limited value. Each syntactic area must be given separate and systematic examination. Knowing the number of errors made under any of the headings below is only the first step; more important is to determine the *pattern* of error, and this is something which cannot be summarized in any simple numerical way. While we leave a place in our classification chart for Stage VI errors, therefore, we must emphasize that the figures it contains have little explanatory value in themselves.

The patterns of error characteristic of this stage we classify under three headings, depending on whether they occur in the Noun Phrase, the Verb Phrase, or affect Clause Structure in some pervasive way. They are listed on the Syntax Profile Chart as minus (−) features. Under the first heading, we pay particular attention to errors in the following grammatical contexts:

(*i*)   There are frequent errors in pronouns at 3½ (e.g. *her doing it, me see*). These are largely eliminated a year later, and during this period there is a corresponding development in the use of reflexives and other pronominal forms not previously used (cf. Webster and Ingram 1972, Huxley 1970, Morehead and Ingram 1973).

---

[14] Error analysis is a widely-used concept in foreign language teaching: see Svartvik 1973, for example. Cf. also Menyuk and Looney 1972, who have a category of 'error types' in their analysis; but their categories—of modification (i.e. changing the transformational operation in sentence structure), substitution (of classes) and omission (when not altering transformational structure) are more abstract than ours. We recognize, however, that the whole concept of 'error' is of doubtful applicability in the context of mother-tongue development in the early years. When we use the term, we mean 'from the point of view of the adult linguistic system'.

Each instance of pronoun error is counted once (under the label *Pron.*) in the procedure described in chapter 5 below.

(*ii*) Determiners have been present since the end of Stage II, but errors in some of the distinctions are still common at $3\frac{1}{2}$ (e.g. confusion over *this* and *that*, or between the articles when used with uncountable nouns). These have largely disappeared a year later. Each error is counted once, under *Det*.

(*iii*) Most of the common irregular noun inflections are stabilized during this Stage, after an earlier period of vacillation between regular and irregular forms. Each error is counted once, under *N irreg*.

(*iv*) Adjective sequence patterns in English display certain fixed tendencies (e.g. one says *a new red chàir*, not **a red new chàir*). We have found that children rarely make mistakes in these sequences. Each sequence containing errors would be counted once, under *Adj seq*.

Under the heading of the Verb Phrase, we note the following:

(*i*) Some auxiliary verbs have been used from around two years (especially *will/won't*, *can/can't*, and *do/don't*): see Morehead and Ingram 1973, Limber 1973. This is another area where syntax is relatively straightforward, but the semantics is complex. Most of the modals appear in Stage VI and come to be widely used, though often with anomalous semantic results, pending the development of the appropriate cognitive operations (e.g. for *ought*, *should*, *must*). Errors such as *he bettern't do it* are eliminated during this Stage. Syntactic errors and semantic errors (where these are determinable) are grouped together in the classification, each instance being counted once, under *Modal*.

(*ii*) This Stage is important for the development and delimitation of the various tense forms and distinctions of aspect, but very little is known about the order of development here, or how these forms tie in with the use of adverbials of time and manner. Some of the forms are present by 3, but mastery of the contrasts does not take place until around now (cf. Herriot 1969), and the use of inappropriate tense or aspect forms is still common before 4. Each error in the syntax or semantics of tense or aspect is counted once, under *Tense*.

(*iii*) Most of the common irregular verb inflections are stabilized during this Stage, as in (*ii*) above. Each error is counted once, under *V irreg*.

Under the heading of Clause Structure, we include:

(*i*) Mistakes in concord are still common at $3\frac{1}{2}$, e.g. *they is, the man are, they hurt himself*, but are generally gone by $4\frac{1}{2}$. (In this area, ability in production often precedes comprehension, cf. Keeney and Wolfe 1972.) Each error is counted once, under *Concord*.

(*ii*) Many adverbs have a restricted position in sentence structure, e.g. *just*, and errors in their use tend to get much less during this stage. Each error is counted once, under *A position*.

(*iii*) Some of the exceptional variations in word order are finally mastered at this Stage, e.g. inversion after negative adverbials, as in *neither did I*. Each error in word order is counted once, under *W. order*.

There is also a category of Other.

System completion, as a label for Stage VI, involves more than the eradication of these 'errors', however. It also involves the development of areas of syntax whose systems of contrasts have been only partly (or not at all) utilized previously (a process which continues into Stage VII). These are listed on the Profile Chart as plus (+) features. In the Noun phrase, we note the following areas:

(i) Initiators (I) are largely developed during this period. Their syntax is relatively simple, but their semantics is more complex, having to do with such matters as quantification and cognitive equivalence, and it is therefore not surprising that their development should be relatively late—after the appropriate cognitive developments have taken place. Each occurrence of an initiator is counted once, any errors in its use being put into the 'Other' category above.

(ii) Coordination patterns (*Coord.*) within the Noun Phrase are of many kinds. A much more adult range of these is developed during this Stage, including some quite lengthy sequences (e.g. lists of objects), appositional structures, and so on. Each instance of a coordinating structure not taken into account at earlier stages (viz. c in Stage IV) is counted once.

In the Verb Phrase, we note one area:

(i) Complex Verb Phrases, e.g. *I should have been able to*, become progressively more adult-like during this period, and errors of word order and selection of inappropriate items tend to disappear. Each string containing more than the sequence already counted at Stage IV is counted once, under *Complex*.

In Clause Structure, two main areas are involved:

(i) The passive voice in its expanded form (e.g. *she's been bitten by a dog*) comes to be used; more complex patterns continue into Stage VII. Each instance of a passive construction of any kind is counted once, under *Passive*.

(ii) More complex patterns of post-verb construction (e.g. *this is ready to eat*, cf. *GCE*, ch. 12) are in evidence, and this continues throughout Stage VII. We include them at this Stage, however, each structure being counted once, under the general heading of complementation (*Complement*).

Other developments are not differentiated, unless they are covered separately by Stage VII. Stage VI structures may therefore be summarized as follows:

(+)			(−)			
NP	*VP*	*Clause*	*NP*		*VP*	*Clause*
Initiator	Complex	Passive	Pron	Adj seq	Modal	Concord
Coord		Complement	Det	N irreg	Tense	A position
					V irreg	W order
Other			Other			

Stage VII: Discourse structure, syntactic comprehension and style

By $4\frac{1}{2}$ the spontaneous speech of children on informal occasions displays fluency and grammatical accuracy in its 'surface' structure. There are few actual grammatical mistakes that can be heard, and while the overall stylistic impression is of a relatively simple and restricted range of expression, it is accordingly not surprising for the impression to be given that the learning of the grammar of the language has been completed by the time a child goes to school. But it would be wrong to conclude this, as a large range of grammatical processes remain to be implemented. They have been little researched, and it may be that further Stages within them will have to be distinguished. For the moment, we operate in terms of three main distinctions.

1   Discourse structure. While the 5-year-old has learned a great deal about sentence structure and function, he still has much to learn about sentence connection—about how a sequence of sentences can be formally interrelated to produce a structured discourse. The following formal syntactic patterns remain to be acquired between 5 and puberty.

(*i*) Sentence-connecting devices, e.g. *however, actually, frankly*. Regardless of the actual meanings involved—some of which are more 'mature' than others—the use of a category of adverbial as a means of relating sentences is not generally found until around age 7. The same applies to most other kinds of connectivity, e.g. the more complex patterns of ellipsis and cross-reference (e.g. . . . . *the other also took one*). Each instance of a connectivity feature of these types is counted once in the classification chart, under *A conn*. Comment clauses (*you know* etc.) are counted separately.

(*ii*) Word-order patterns controlling the distribution of emphasis are also learned relatively late (e.g. *John Smith his name is*), as well as more subtle exceptions to the rules of word order previously learned (e.g. *hardly had I gone* . . . , where the SV order is reversed). Under this heading also one would place clause sequences introduced by *it* or *there* (e.g. *it's John who said he couldn't come*), and most of the other complex embeddings described by *GCE* in chapter 14. We count *it* and *there* patterns separately, but all other variations in normal clause order for purposes of emphasis are grouped together under *Emphatic Order*.

(*iii*) The use of intonation to control the relationships between the various parts of a sentence is also learned, e.g. *John gave the book to Jim and hě gave one to hìm* (i.e. Jim gave one to John also). Mastery of this use of intonation is still going on at age 9 (cf. Cruttenden 1974), but the overall pattern of development is unclear, and we have not as yet given this area any quantitative analysis.

In addition to these discourse-sensitive features, Stage VII also concludes the learning of irregular forms of nouns, verbs etc. One often finds 7- or 8-year-olds who are still having trouble with the occasional irregular form, e.g. *tooken* instead of *took*. Also, the rule governing the two types of comparison (*prettier* v. *more interesting*) takes some while to be properly learned. Mistakes in the sequence of tenses and other subordinate/main clause relations also come to be sorted out during this Stage. (See further Hunt 1970, Amidon and Carey 1972.)

2   Syntactic comprehension. The emphasis here may be summarized by saying that just because a 5-year-old can produce a syntactic pattern, this is no guarantee that he has understood what he has said. This point is familiar in relation to vocabulary, where knowing the word but not the meaning is a feature common in young (as well as not-so-young) children. But the point seems to have been neglected for syntax. Carol Chomsky (1969) has illustrated the kind of syntactic awareness that needs to develop.[15] The two sentences

(*1*) John is eager to please   (*2*) John is easy to please

have an identical 'surface' appearance: S V C. But we as adults know that in (*1*) John is the person who is doing the pleasing (i.e. he is the 'real' Subject of the Verb; he is doing the action), whereas in (*2*) he is the person who is being pleased (he is the 'real' Object of the Verb; he is receiving the action). We can predict that as the majority of sentences that young children encounter are of type (*1*)— that is, the Subject goes before the Verb, and does the action—it is the 'exceptional' cases, like (*2*), which will cause trouble. Children will presumably try to use (*2*) as if it meant (*1*), and this is what we find. 5-year-olds, given a situation with a blindfolded doll, and asked 'Is the doll easy to see?', Chomsky found tend to answer 'No, it can't.' 7-year-olds, on the other hand, are on the whole able to respond appropriately. There are many such distinctions where two sentences have widely different interpretations but identical structures, e.g. *Ask him what to do/Tell him what to do, I told John to come/I promised John to come*, and it does take children quite a while to sort these out. Another example would be the semantically more complex conjunctions, e.g. *since, unless, although*, which can continue to be confused with *and* as late as 9 years old. In Stage VII, then, an important development is in the child becoming aware that the meaning, or 'deep' analysis of a sentence is not always obvious from a consideration of its 'surface' pattern. Things are not always what they seem. This new dimension to language analysis may also be seen in the child's increased ability to detect ambiguity, and to use it himself, in puns and riddles—a notable characteristic of young children's comics and Christmas Annuals after about age 6 (cf. Shultz and Pilon 1973). A pun is a play on words, i.e. two interpretations for a single utterance; it accordingly fits well with the distinction between deep and surface structure just referred to.

3   Style. As soon as the child goes to school he is put into regular contact with speech norms that may be unfamiliar to him. Previously, most children have had relatively little direct contact with language from outside the immediate family circle. Now they find themselves in contact with new accents, vocabularies (e.g. words for toiletry) and grammatical patterns. The existence of stylistic variety is even more evident as they learn to read, and as they become aware of the notion of standards of correctness, both in reading/writing and in speaking/listening. This period of sociolinguistic and personal development is complex and little studied.

[15] It makes an interesting theoretical question whether these problems are primarily of syntax or semantics. Both factors are involved. See Cromer (1970) and Cambon and Sinclair (1974) for discussion of the methodological problems raised by Chomsky's approach.

All we wish to point out here is that syntax is inevitably affected—new structures appear which have a purely stylistic role; children develop likes and dislikes in their ways of speaking (and listening); their conscious awareness of features of language (such as sentence, noun, verb) develops along lines laid down by the school, and this may affect their own linguistic ability (cf. Hart 1975); and the first hints of a stylistic idiosyncrasy in syntax emerge. Stylistic development is something which lasts long after puberty, of course. Some say it is a process which never ends. But before puberty, it becomes evident in the greater flexibility and range of structures used by the child, and it is this which justifies its brief mention at this Stage.

As with Stage VI, it is not possible as yet to classify the developments of Stage VII in a precise, exhaustive, numerical way. We cite the above areas as a focus for discussion and analysis, and hope that they are suggestive of guidelines for practical use. The main Stage VII patterns are mentioned on the classification summary chart below, but only for the sake of completeness.

There has been repeated mention of puberty, especially during the last few paragraphs. Its significance for us is that we feel that it is with puberty that the period of syntactic development comes to an end. After this, the language-learning ability changes dramatically, and spontaneous learning is more a matter of developing stylistic skills, writing and reading abilities, and vocabulary. The evidence for seeing puberty as a linguistically significant stage is various, and of varying degrees of cogency. The main evidence is from pathological studies and is summarized by Lenneberg (1967, 142ff.). For example, the consequences of undergoing a left hemispherectomy (the surgical removal of the left hemisphere of the brain, which is where the centre of speech is traditionally supposed to lie) depend upon the age at which the original insult (such as a tumour) was incurred. Before puberty, if the child had a lesion (regardless of side), speech function was eventually confined to the healthy hemisphere, so that when the diseased hemisphere was removed (either then, or later in life), there was no aphasia. On the other hand, patients who acquired their lesion in later life, and who underwent hemispherec-tomy, had permanent aphasic symptoms if the operation was done on the left side, with negligible spontaneous regeneration of language. Other evidence is less direct: one may compare the performance of 'dysphasic' children and dysphasic adults and show that in terms of their reaction to remedial procedures, their response patterns are widely different;[16] one may compare the abilities of pre- and post-puberty children in learning a foreign language; one may analyse the syntactic characteristics of spontaneous speech before and after puberty, to show differences in the range of structures used; and so on. All in all, the evidence is considerable for viewing puberty as marking the end of a critical period for syntactic develop-ment. Certainly, for our purposes, we take our syntactic procedure no further.

[16] See further ch. 6. We differ from Lenneberg who, in our view, overstates the difference in respect of syntax. An adult aphasic, when his symptoms subside, does not display, according to Lenneberg, 'a gradual emergence of the more complex grammatical constructions' (144). We find some evidence that he does.

We can now summarize the various Stages described by bringing the patterns together into a single Classification Chart. It is this which provides the developmental component necessary for implementing our syntactic procedure. The chart is given on p. 85.

A final word about chronological norms. It seems to be the case that almost all the child-language research has been carried out on the children of parents who fall within the upper ranges of the various socioeconomic scales. It may well be, then, that the chronological norms cited above are likely to be high when compared with children from lower socioeconomic backgrounds—or so, these days, we are led to believe. Whatever the facts, we advocate caution and flexibility in using these age ranges, and would suggest that each age range be viewed as a mean. A spread of ±6 months is quite tolerable within the notion of 'normal age range', when varied populations of children are taken into account; but we cannot be more precise about this until standardization studies come to be done (see Postscript, below).

A	**Unanalysed**					**Problematic**			
	1 Unintelligible		2 Symbolic Noise		3 Deviant	1 Incomplete		2 Ambiguous	

B	**Responses**				Normal Response						Abnormal			
				Repet-itions	Elliptical Major				Full Major	Minor	Struc-tural	∅	Prob-lems
	Stimulus Type		Totals		1	2	3	4					
		Questions											
		Others											

C	**Spontaneous**			Others	

		Minor				*Social*	*Stereotypes*	*Problems*	
Stage I (0;9–1;6)	Sentence Type	**Major**					Sentence Structure		
		Excl.	*Comm.*	*Quest.*			*Statement*		
			·V·	·Q·	·V·	·N·	Other	Problems	

				Conn.	Clause		Phrase		Word
Stage II (1;6–2;0)		V X	Q X		SV	V C/O	DN	VV	-ing
					S C/O	A X	Adj N	V part	pl
					Neg X	Other	NN	Int X	
							PrN	Other	-ed
Stage III (2;0–2;6)		V X Y	Q X Y		X + S:NP	X + V:VP	X + C/O:NP	X + A:AP	
		let X Y	VS		SVC/O	VC/OA	D Adj N	Cop	-en
		do X Y			SVA	VO_dO_i	Adj Adj N	Aux	
					Neg X Y	Other	Pr DN	Pron	3s
							N Adj N	Other	gen
Stage IV (2;6–3;0)		÷ S	QVS		XY + S:NP	XY + V:VP	XY + C/O:NP	XY + A:AP	n't
			Q X Y Z		SVC/OA	AAXY	N Pr NP	Neg V	'cop
					SVO_dO_i	Other	Pr D Adj N	Neg X	'aux
							cX	2 Aux	
							XcX	Other	
Stage V (3;0–3;6)		how	tag	and	Coord. 1 1 +		Postmod. 1 1 + clause		-est
				c	Subord. 1 1 +				-er
		what		s	Clause: S		Postmod. 1 + phrase		-ly
				Other	Clause: C/O				
					Comparative				

	(+)			(−)				
	NP	*VP*	*Clause*	*NP*		*VP*	*Clause*	
Stage VI (3;6–4;6)	Initiator	Complex	Passive	Pron	Adj seq	Modal	Concord	
	Coord		Complement	Det	N irreg	Tense	A position	
						V irreg	W order	
	Other			Other				

	Discourse		*Syntactic Comprehension*	
Stage VII (4;6 +)	A Connectivity	it		
	Comment Clause	·there	*Style*	
	Emphatic Order	Other		

Total No. Sentences	Mean No. Sentences Per Turn	Mean Sentence Length

© D. Crystal, P. Fletcher, M. Garman, 1975 University of Reading

Profile chart: developmental stages

5

A language assessment, remediation and screening procedure (LARSP)

We are now in a position to use the information about normal and adult syntax in order to formulate a specific procedure for remedial work. For convenience of reference, we shall label this LARSP, as in the title to this chapter. In the various stages of its implementation, the procedure is similar to others currently in use (e.g. Engler *et al.* 1973). Seven stages are recognized: (*i*) sampling, (*ii*) transcription, (*iii*) grammatical analysis, (*iv*) structure count, (*v*) pattern evaluation, (*vi*) statement of remedial goals, and (*vii*) statement of remedial procedures. In this chapter, we deal with points (*i*) to (*iv*).

(i) Sampling

Obtaining the best possible sample of data from P is obviously fundamental to the whole exercise, and we rely on sampling of free conversational interaction as part of our routine procedure, as opposed to other methods of eliciting data. Formal testing (in sentence frames etc.) gives little indication of spontaneous ability, and is very selective. We agree with Lee and Canter (1971, 316), who say 'a clinical procedure such as the analysis of a speech sample may yield more useful information to a clinician than does traditional testing.' We have no theoretical objection to the use of imitation tasks as a means of discovering information about linguistic ability, and find valuable the approach of Slobin and Welsh (1968), and subsequent work (e.g. Jordan and Robinson 1972, Miller 1973, Rodd and Braine 1970), which concludes concerning elicited imitation tasks that 'in repeating a sentence, one must filter it through one's own productive system' (Slobin and Welsh, see p. 490). Cf. Menyuk and Looney (1972, 265), who argue that normal children's (3- to 7-year-olds, in their work) repetitions 'reflect their level of grammatical competence.' But devising a scheme for use in assessment and remediation needs a wider range of data than imitation tasks can provide—especially when sentence length gets longer than a certain point. Systems like Lee's (1969) are of use as a quick screening test, but for more complex assessment, the range of imitation patterns to be elicited would need to be very large. We therefore orient our procedure as far as possible to the analysis of samples of natural conversation under certain conditions (see below).

Three important considerations must influence the selection of any speech sample: characteristics of the recording situation, the amount of data required, and the range of sentence patterns considered analysable. For our purposes, all these factors are decided bearing in mind the need for comparability of normal samples with those it is feasible to obtain in the clinical situation. It is no good demanding that 500 utterances, or an hour's worth of data, or a sample of a child–child interaction as the desideratum, when the typical clinical situation is adult–child, with an average of 30–45 minutes per session before the child gets tired, and so on. We have therefore looked first to see what kind of samples are most readily elicitable in clinical situations, and placed our normal children and adults in the same situation. With this in mind, our initial decision was to measure all samples in terms of time rather than number of utterances, as this is a measure more readily appreciated and adhered to when Ts provide us with samples from their sessions. We have selected samples of 30 minutes' duration, which avoids most problems of fatigue with Ps, and is a realistic request for Ts to conform to.

In normal children in Stages I to V, 30 minutes in the situations described below produces between 100 and 200 sentences. This may be compared with traditional sample sizes which, while being very variable (see the discussion in Darley and Moll 1960, Minifie *et al.* 1963 and Shriner and Sherman 1967), tend to be much smaller. Fifty utterances is the classical sample size in this field: see for example McCarthy 1930 (32), 1954, Hahn 1948, Templin 1957, Brannon and Murry 1966, Lee and Canter 1971. Some scholars however use much less (as little as 15, in the case of Schneiderman (1955) and, more recently, Griffith and Miner (1969)), and most these days use 100: Menyuk (1964), Brown (1973), Longhurst and Schrandt (1973), and also Nice (1925). Between 100 and 200 is used by Morehead and Ingram (1973), and Ingram (1972c). Morehead (1972, 5) thinks in terms of 500, which is indeed 'large'. Engler *et al.* (1973) use an open-ended technique, recording for 5/10 minutes, and aiming for 75–100 utterances which 'should be sufficient to begin with' (194). Limber (1973) uses two 30-minute samples, one with parents, and one with the analyst. There is some difference of opinion as to *which* part of a recording the sample should be taken from, e.g. Tyack (1972a) takes her utterances from the first section of a sample, Brown (1973, 54) from the second page of the transcription onwards, Lee and Canter (1971) with the last 50 utterances (to avoid any warm-up period, and to recognize 'the possibility that pictures and stories might elicit more sophisticated language than free play' (334)). Minifie *et al.* (1963) argue that the means of three 50-utterance samples are adequate, and provide reasonable temporal reliability. Darley and Moll (1960) claim that a single measure of 50 gives optimum predictability and reliability, and they accept that adequacy depends on aims, and the kind of precision needed.

The 30-minute samples which we use are obtained from two periods of continuous taping, usually from a single recording session. The first period, in the case of children, involves approximately 15 minutes of conversational interaction in an unstructured, free play situation (using toys[1] which do not make too much noise). The interviewer (normally the parent or regular guardian, but it could be T, if the child knows him well) should play alone with the child in what he considers to be

---

[1] Not books or pictures, unless T has no alternative. We find that many Ps who do not respond to pictures will do so for toys, and we therefore use the latter as far as possible. In this respect, our procedure differs from that of Engler *et al.* (1973), who use pictures alone.

a natural, appropriate way. If the child stays fairly quiet, the session can be turned into a prompted dialogue (asking the child what he's doing, what's happening etc.). The second period involves approximately 15 minutes of dialogue on some aspect of the child's experience not to do with the immediate play-situation, e.g. asking about family, holidays, school, or the imagined biography of the toys.[2] In both situations, it is up to the adult to decide whether the time is ripe for recording. To decide this, he must make full use of his intuitive knowledge of the child's ability, as he must after the recording session is over, in judging whether the sample obtained was reasonably representative. No one can be precise about such matters, but if the child's close contacts .are agreed in their intuitive assessments that a session was 'average', 'quieter than usual' etc., this information can be of considerable value in assessing the applicability of any analysis. We usually suggest that any opening exchanges are not part of the recorded sample (e.g. when P comes to visit T), as linguistically they are in many ways atypical of any subsequent utterance; but apart from this we do not constrain the parent's/T's judgement in any way. We do however insist that the samples be as unstructured as possible, and discuss with parents or T beforehand the importance of not pressuring the child to produce more utterances than one would normally expect him. If T is doing the recording, it is important that he does not let his remediation habits colour the dialogue too much (e.g. instinctively correcting P's utterance, or providing structured prompts). In some clinical situations, of course, it is impossible to elicit anything from P without a high degree of structuring, but this we see as a last resort.[3]

Our sampling emphasis is therefore very similar to that recommended by Lee and Canter (1971), whose recipe is to take 50 'complete, different, consecutive, intelligible, nonecholalic sentences elicited from a child in conversation with an adult, using stimulus materials . . .' (317). But we do make a number of different decisions at various places.

(a)   *Complete.* Lee and Canter mean 'at least a noun and a verb in subject–predicate relationship' (317) (though they count imperatives as complete). We see two problems in this. We often do not know what counts as a fragment in their examples (e.g. why the parenthesized section of (*Over there, but*) *it's too far away* is considered fragmentary). Secondly, we feel that this restriction omits too much information of potential remedial value. Not only are essential facts about Stages I and II lost, but it should be remembered in addition that fragments often provide important leads. In a sense, T is not interested in knowing what P can do well, but in what he cannot do, and in the boundary area between the two. It is in this boundary area that fragments will tend to occur, as P begins a sentence, gets into difficulties, and leaves it. Knowing the number and range of fragmentary con-

---

[2] This division may be compared with Morehead and Ingram (1973), who make three divisions (free play with adults, eliciting utterances using toys, and eliciting using books), and Lee and Canter (1971), who also use a threefold division, with toys, talking about a set of pictures, and telling a story (Three Bears) using pictures.

[3] A certain amount of automatic structuring by T in fact characterizes our first samples in the case studies reported in chapters 7 and 8.

structions compared to the number of 'complete' ones is, we find, an important statistic in any assessment.[4]

(b) *Different* is an important notion, 'to avoid overused stereotypes' (318). But it is important also not to lose this information, as variation in the frequency with which P repeats himself may be a significant index of progress, or lack of it.

(c) *Consecutive:* 'to avoid selecting only high-scoring utterances' (318). We also insist on continuous recording.

(d) *Intelligible.* Lee and Canter here mean that utterances ought not to be penalized for articulatory difficulty, and should be reasonably self-contained. T should not have to read in too much to make sense of it. Sentences are excluded if their potentially scorable parts cannot be understood.[5] We accept the distinction between intelligible and unintelligible, but we retain the information about the number of unintelligible utterances, as this can provide an indication of progress.

(e) *Nonecholalic.* Likewise here, we wish to distinguish utterances that are 'not spontaneously formulated' (318), but we do not wish to exclude them from our sample, and a note about the amount of echolalia is incorporated in our data classification chart.

The main difference between our sampling and that of most of the authors we have read is that we have not regularized our data in any way. Whatever turns up in the 30 minutes we must find a place for in our classification, which aims to be exhaustive.

Exactly the same factors need to be borne in mind in investigating the speech of disordered adults, except that (a) visual materials can be used as a routine eliciting technique, and (b) the analyst's own intuition is available as a normative base, in addition to any 30-minute samples he may have available.

Lastly, under this heading, while we accept that any sample is undoubtedly limited in the amount of generalization it can stimulate, we do not see these limitations as being a cause of fundamental concern, when it comes to comparing performances of different children. We do not believe in the view that it is possible to 'match' samples in some theoretically absolute way, with all variables controlled (cf. Muma 1973b). Such matching demands are beyond the bounds of any known procedures. As long as the main biases in sampling are guarded against, by being aware of the factors referred to above, we feel that this is all that can reasonably be done.

No one knows the extent to which nonlinguistic variables influence speech norms and interact to produce group syntactic profiles. It is therefore important

---

[4] Moreover, a single instance of a pattern is sufficient to warrant the ascription of that pattern to a Stage on the classification chart.

The chart makes no theoretical assumptions about productivity, which is a separate decision, to be made at a later stage. We see a danger in bringing in these considerations at the sampling stage, as do, say, Morehead and Ingram (1973), who want each linguistic structure to occur at least twice 'to be considered part of the child's productive system' (234).

[5] Cf. Muma (1971), who also includes only unproblematic sentences. His sample contains the initial 60 +T-units—a +T-unit being one that presents no transcription/segmentation difficulty.

that we obtain as much information as current theory suggests may be relevant to establish group norms. Each recording is thus accompanied by a data sheet on which social, family etc. information is given (see Appendix A). For normal children, the relevant questions are as follows:

Background data

1   Date of birth
2   Sex
3   Age and sex of sibs
4   Age of father and mother
5   Where living now
6   Occupation of father and mother
7   Does either parent have a noticeable regional accent?
8   Have either any obvious speech/hearing impediment?
9   Child's medical history: normal birth? any long stays in hospital? any major disability or illness?
10   Any school/nursery/creche etc. attendance? (state what kind and how long)
11   Is the child in regular contact with other adults at home? (state relationship)
12   Does the child have any contact with languages other than English? (state which)
13   Give any psychological testing scores which may be available
14   Any other information considered relevant

Recording data

1   Where did the recording take place?
2   Date of recording.
3   Anything abnormal in the child's general behaviour, health etc.?
4   Anything abnormal in the situation, which may have influenced the way he reacted, and which is not obvious from the tape?

For disordered Ps, a more detailed account is taken, paying particular attention to medical history and the details of the therapy session. This is given in full in Appendix B. For adults, we use a set of questions similar to the child's above, but in addition we ask for a Communicative History form to be completed by P's next-of-kin as an aid to semantic interpretation of his utterances, and later, as a source of suggestions for conversation topics to use or avoid. This form is given in full in Appendix C.

(ii)   Transcription

It is easy to underestimate the amount of skill required in order to make a good transcription. By 'good transcription' we mean a visual record of the taped language used in a situation, which can take the place of the original recording accurately and unambiguously. With a satisfactory transcription, it should be unnecessary for the analyst to need to refer back to the tape to clarify or clear up points of uncertainty. It is therefore essential, in our view, that adequate prosodic cues are incorporated into the transcription to permit an accurate recapitulation of the movement and organization of the speech flow, and we have already described the contrasts which we have found to be an obligatory minimum (see chapter 3). Marking intonation and pause, however, is a specialist skill. Even listening to speech on tape to provide a basic transcription of the words used is something of a skill, which improves dramatically with practice. The transcription, therefore, is something for which the analyst has to be responsible, and which he needs to check his ability to do (cf. Shriner 1969). It is not a task which can be casually assigned to an audiotypist, unless the individual concerned has been given some prior training. Much of the American work uses typists routinely (e.g. Engler *et al.* 1973), but in no way can their output be considered an adequate transcription.[6] Pause, intonation and rhythm *must* be marked, as we have already said, if a realistic account of the P's confidence, hesitancy, ability to structure his utterances, ability to complete utterances, and so on, is to be obtained—as also for the definition of utterance in the first place (as in Longhurst and Schrandt 1973).

Where the linguist *does* need help in the transcription is in the early stages of interpreting the situation as reflected in the taped record. Any sample of data must be gone through as soon as possible after it was obtained by the person involved in the interaction, and notes or a rough transcription provided of those parts of the recording which would be unintelligible or obscure to anyone who had not been present in the situation. There will always be difficulties of this kind, and unless one is in the fortunate position of having an adult observer behind a one-way screen, who can make notes as the session proceeds, or a video record, there is no alternative but for the participating adult to listen through the tape and add as much background information as he can. Examples of difficulty for the outside listener would be: (*a*) immature articulation which is not glossed on the tape; (*b*) family slang and other nonstandard words and phrases; (*c*) personal information about P, e.g. if a name of a brother is used; and (*d*) glossing utterances that are dependent on some situational event, e.g. *hello* to someone waving through the window; *fall down* said after a brick had fallen over. We have found that the best time to draw up this commentary is immediately after the session. If it is not made within a few hours, its completeness and reliability diminish considerably.

Transcriptions for LARSP are made using a standard sheet with left- and right-hand margins. Reference information (Name of P, Recording Date, Session Number, Page of Transcript, and Index Number of Tape) is given across the top of the page. In the right-hand margin is placed suggestions about alternative readings, any additional information about the quality of the recording at a given point (e.g. 'bad aeroplane noise', 'child moves away from microphone'), information about any speech characteristics that the basic transcription does not provide

---

[6] Engler *et al.* have some pause marks, but they are not graded, and no information is given about intonation.

but which are felt to be important at a given point (e.g. 'very irritated', 'husky voice'), and any of the analyst's impressions as he goes through the material for the first time (e.g. 'NB tense form'). The only information in the left-hand margin is the initials used to mark the change of speaker, usually T and P, with others being used depending on the number of participants. As regards the transcription, each change of speaker commences a new line. Also, within each speaker we adopt the convention that each new sentence begins a new line. (The aim of this is to enable us to obtain from a transcript an immediate impression of the quantity of P's utterance in the session compared with T's, and whether or not P is responding to T's utterances. It also simplifies the sentence-counting procedure later.) Other features of the transcription are:

(*a*)   ( ) is used to enclose uninterpretable speech; it is either left blank, or may include an indication of the shape of the utterance, e.g. (*2 syllables*). A stretch of transcription enclosed in parenthesis indicates that its status is really only a guess at what was on the tape, e.g. (*everyone know*) *that it's red.*

(*b*)   A question-mark before a word indicates some doubt about the transcriptional accuracy of that word, often due to a disagreement between two listeners, e.g. *leading ?the dog.*

(*c*)   Any nonlinguistic vocal information is written in to the transcript at the appropriate point, e.g. *laughs, yawns.*

(*d*)   If the participants overlap in their speech, the point of overlap is marked with an asterisk, e.g.

T   so he 'said he *will
P   *'he will còme/

A brief or incomplete utterance which does not interrupt the speaker's flow is indicated at the point it occurs using double parentheses, e.g.

T   so he 'said he (('I want)) would 'stay lónger/
T   'after a 'while ((yès/)) he 'went hòme/.

(*e*)   Capital letters are not needed at the beginnings of sentences, but they are kept for ease of reading in the case of proper names, abbreviations, and the pronoun *I.*

A sample page of transcription follows. It is of a 16-year-old boy from a special school.

Tape No. 2	*Name PD*	*Rec. date 20.9.73*	*Session 1 Page 3*
T	'what do we 'have hére/ —		*shows picture*
P	er — —		
T	'what's thìs/ —		
P	er — — màn/		
T	it îs a 'man/ îsn't it/ .		
	'what's the 'man doìng/		
P	?'leading the dòg/		

Tape No. 2	Name PD	Rec. date 20.9.73	Session 1 Page 3

T	yês/ a 'man with a dòg/ . 'where are they gòing/	
P	for a wàlk/	
T	for a wâlk/ — for a 'walk a'cross the fîeld/ — do you 'like that pícture/ is 'that a níce 'picture/	
P	pīcture/	
T	and 'what's hère/	*shows another*
P	màn/ màn/	*picture*
T	'what's thàt man 'doing/	
P	'smoking a cìgarette/	
T	'smoking a 'cigarètte/ yès/ he ìs/ ìsn't he/ do you 'like fóotball/ — —	*picks up book*
	you were 'playing 'football when I sàw you/ wèren't you/ — — you were 'playing 'football with the bòys/ — — — that 'book's all abòut fóotball/ ìsn't it/ — 'let's have a lòok in it/ — — 'what's thìs/ hère/	
P	a bàll/	
T	it ís/ — 'what kìnd of a 'ball/	
P	yèllow/	
T	'somebody kìcked that báll/ *dìdn't they/	
P	*yès/	
T	whò 'kicked that 'ball/ 'which màn 'kicked that 'ball/	
P	?this 'man 'kicked that bàll/	*NB unexpected*
T	he dîd/ yês/ — — —	*inton. tonic*

As a general rule, in the context of our research, all transcripts are checked by two analysts working independently, and points of disagreement noted accordingly.

(iii) Grammatical analysis

Each of P's sentences is analysed using the apparatus of chapter 3. There are many possible ways of working through the data, and the investigator may be left to work out the method which he personally finds most convenient. The following guidelines, which we ourselves follow, may be helpful. We work through the data in repeated scans, eight in all. In each scan, the data are examined from a specific point of view.

Scan 1. This determines the range of sentences which cannot be analysed, or which raise problems which have to be deferred until later in the analysis. Under the first heading, we include three categories of utterance. (*a*) The sentence or utterance is wholly unintelligible (or a sufficient amount of it is to make assignment of a grammatical description impossible). (*b*) Symbolic noise (such as imitations of ambulance sirens) are taken separately. Hesitation noises are not counted at all. (*c*) Deviant sentences (see p. 28), which we want to keep separate from the expected sentence types. If we were uncertain of the deviant status of a sentence, we would analyse it in the normal way.

Under the second heading, there are also two utterance categories. (*a*) The sentence is incomplete (for whatever reason), this usually being clear from the incomplete prosody. Unfinished sentences may be referred to later in the analysis, as 'extra' information to support or reject some generalization that may have been made on the basis of the complete sentences; but any such use must be made with caution. However, partials due to someone having a repeated go at starting a sentence (e.g. the first three words of *he . he said . he said he'd come/* are ignored in the analysis. (*b*) We also defer analysis of the second category, ambiguous sentences. Here we mean sentences which could receive two (or more) quite different but equally plausible syntactic interpretations, and it is unclear from all available (structural or situational) information which is correct. To choose one arbitrarily would be of little help. These cases are best placed on one side and left unanalysed until after the rest of the analysis has taken place. There may then be internal evidence to suggest that analysis A is the only one P seems capable of, and the ambiguous sentences can then be included in the structure count (see below). If there is no such evidence, the ambiguity must be allowed to stand, and the proportion of syntactically ambiguous sentences remaining in a sample at the end of the analysis can be of great interest.[7]

The first scan, then, tries to ensure that subsequent scans will be as unproblematic as possible, so that a rapid and continuous analysis can be made. They are not taken further into account in the analysis of sections B, C and the Stages. Even if one is only slightly dubious about a sentence, it is worth putting it into the 'problematic file' for a more leisurely examination later, if this should prove necessary. Our aim, it should be emphasized, is to get an analysis done as quickly as possible. It may well be that the description of the clear sentence patterns will be sufficient for our purposes, so that the dubious patterns will never need to be consulted. If they are left mixed in with the clear patterns, however, the whole procedure can become extremely time-consuming.

Scan 2. This establishes the proportion of spontaneous to response sentences in the sample, and provides an analysis of the type of response. This distinction

---

[7] Note that a sentence may be structurally ambiguous at only one point or one grammatical level, e.g. *The man was killed by the tree* (= near the tree or by means of the tree?) is ambiguous in terms of clause structure only. It is more convenient to put the *whole* sentence on one side, however, dealing with it separately later.

provides basic information of obvious significance in remedial work:[8] to what extent is P spontaneously using language, and to what extent will he speak only when spoken to—and if the latter, what kind of response is he most likely to come out with? It is normally no problem to distinguish spontaneous from response utterances. It may however sometimes be a problem deciding which sentence P's utterance can be said to respond to. Generally it is the immediately preceding sentence T has produced. In some cases, however, P can only be responding to an earlier sentence than T's last, e.g.

T   'where's the cár/ — — can you sée it/
P   'in the ròad/ .

It is sometimes unclear which of a number of preceding sentences P is in fact responding to, and in such cases we place a mark in the Problem box, referred to below. It should be noted, however, that in such cases pause-marks may help to indicate the main stimulus sentence, by showing that T has waited for a response before trying an alternative cue. Brief vocalizations used by T while P is speaking (e.g. *mhm*, *yes*) are ignored in classifying P's response types: they would be treated as stimuli only when used in isolation, during a pause, as a specific indication that P should continue. (When P uses these vocalizations while T is speaking, they are of course counted—under 'minor responses' and 'social'.)

Responses. These are classified according to the type of stimulus sentence. We have generally found it useful to distinguish *Question* stimuli from all other kinds, not making subdivisions within the latter (e.g. whether T's prompt sentence was a statement, command, or exclamation of some kind) on the grounds that the various categories are not sufficiently frequent to warrant the effort. The total number of 'Questions' vs. 'Others' is included before these headings in section B. Nor on the chart do we distinguish within stimulus type the various possibilities in the remediation context, e.g. prompt questions, elicited imitation questions etc. (see chapter 6). The various possible response patters are subclassified, however, in the following way:

(*a*)   *Normal response* type. There are three main syntactic processes whereby one may respond normally in standard English.

(*i*) One may answer with a full major sentence, e.g. Q. *Where's the book?* A. *It's in the box.*

(*ii*) One may answer with an elliptical major sentence, e.g. Q. *Where's the book?* A. *In the box.* In clear cases of ellipsis, it must be recalled (cf. chapter 3), it is always possible to give an exact specification of the omitted elements of structure by referring to the structure of the previous sentence. (This is what distinguished ellipsis from incomplete sentences, discussed above, where it is impossible to relate a piece of utterance to any of the language in the surrounding context.) Thus in the sentence *Where's John?* the answer *In the garden* involves the elision of SV. It is important to know how far P can take previous sentence structure for granted in this way. The significance of normal redundancy is often ignored in

---

[8] It is a basic division in Morehead and Ingram 1973, for example.

clinical procedures, where 'full' answers are demanded and rated higher than elliptical ones (cf. p. 13), and we are strongly opposed to such an emphasis. There are however many possible elliptical patterns, some quite infrequent. We therefore classify elliptical responses into four main types: whether the ellipsis has resulted in the whole or part of one element of structure remaining (S, V, C, O, or A); whether two elements remain (SV, VO, VC etc.); whether three elements remain (e.g. VOA, SVA); and (less commonly) whether four or more elements remain (e.g. VOAA).[9]

(iii) One may answer with a Minor Sentence, usually yes, no, mhm etc.

(b)   Abnormal response type. There are two subtypes. One is zero response (symbolized as ∅), where some response is clearly expected but is not provided. This might usefully be subclassified in terms of stimulus structures, if a sample showed a high frequency, but we do not carry out such a classification as a routine. The second type is structural deviance, i.e. a syntactic pattern is used which is not a possible match for the syntax of the stimulus sentence, e.g. Q. Where are you going? A. Yes. or Q. Is that a dog? A. In the road. Note the fact that the answer may be highly motivated by the situation—the dog might be in the road, in this example—makes this nonetheless an abnormal response on syntactic grounds.

(c)   Repetitions. This is a broad category which includes any of P's sentences where there is cause to think that P is doing no more than repeating all or part of T's structure. Thus this category subsumes all that is traditionally called echolalia (automatic repetition of previous speech) as well as elicited imitations ('say bus' etc.), and repeats of one or more words even where comprehension might be said to be present, e.g. T. It's a bus. P. Bus. We do not include under this heading responses to 'forced alternative' questions (see chapter 6), e.g. Is it a blue bus or a red one?, as here the element of choice in the reponse is still present.[10] All repetitions are analysed in terms of sections B, C and the Stages. The number in the repetitions box should therefore always be referred to before confident statements about spontaneity of language use are made.

(d)   Problems. Under this heading we include any case where allocation to one of the above categories is uncertain, or where there is some doubt as to whether the sentence was spontaneous. Placing dubious cases here, rather than under the

---

[9] An interesting theoretical point arises in relation to ellipsis. A child who says ball in answer to the question What did daddy kick? may or may not have an SVO pattern in his production, but we take it by the appropriateness of his reponse that he has such a pattern in his comprehension. We do not however know whether making this assumption at Stages before III is reasonable. Nor do we have data on developmental norms of children's ability to elide, but we do feel that statements such as the following are premature: 'We expect that ellipted utterances will begin to occur later than complete utterances' (Dever and Bauman 1971, 30).

[10] The distinction between echoing and imitation is not one that can be made on the basis of isolated examples. The terms refer to alternative strategies P may be following overall, and so a decision on whether a particular response by P is echoed or imitated will depend not just on that response but on the overall picture from the whole sample. The usual interpretation of echoing is a consistent repetition by P of the final item or items from the stimulus sentence. The implication is that the child is performing the absolute minimum of language processing on what he hears. Imitation, for our purposes, is a strategy by which P takes some part of an utterance from T and reproduces it himself. In some cases he will produce the final item he has heard, in others not.

heading of 'spontaneous' below, is an arbitrary decision, but one which avoids the danger of overestimating P's spontaneous ability.

The total number of *all* responses to Questions/Others, excluding zero, is included under the heading 'Total'. This figure then allows an immediate comparison to be made between stimulus sentences used and responses obtained, e.g. 30 QUESTIONS 21 (i.e. of 30 question-stimuli, 9 were either zero or unanalysed, cf. Section A).

Spontaneous sentences. The main division made under this heading is to distinguish self-repetitions from novel sentences. For example, where exactly the same sentence is used more than once within an utterance, it would be overestimating P's ability to count each instance as a novel instance of the syntactic pattern. A separate tally of repeated sentences is therefore made. *Any* change in the sentence, no matter how slight (e.g. even if it is only in the intonation), provides grounds for taking the two sentences as independent.[11]

Novel sentences are not further subclassified, with the exception of one-element sentences which are clearly elliptical (cf. p. 50), e.g. *Lunch?*, *Ready?* It would be unrealistic to classify an adult's use of these along with the one-element sentences of Stage I, where ellipsis would be an absurd overestimate of the child's syntactic ability. By the end of Stage II, though, it seems reasonable to attribute some awareness of ellipsis to the child. Accordingly we classify all spontaneous major elliptical sentences with two or more elements in the usual way between Stages II and VII. The same applies to all complete major sentences listed under the heading of Spontaneous (Other). Spontaneous 'comments', made while T is speaking (e.g. *mhm*), are also counted under Other in section C.

We may now summarize the classification procedure on the second scan as follows:

B	Responses				Normal Response						Abnormal		
					Elliptical Major				Full		Struc-		Prob-
	Stimulus Type	Totals	Repet-itions	1	2	3	4		Major	Minor	tural	Ø	lems
	Questions												
	Others												
C	Spontaneous			Others									

Scan 3. Here the data are analysed sentence by sentence at the level of sentence connectivity: each type is tabulated and a count made. In most cases of language disability, this can be done fairly quickly, as there will be little connectivity present.

---

[11] We do not, however, count as repetition the repeated use of a single word or phrase within a sentence, when this is obviously due to hesitation, or some such case, e.g. *I'm going to . to the cinema* is analysed as *I'm going to the cinema*.

Scan 4. Sentence structure is analysed, in terms of coordination, subordination etc. This too generally takes little time.

Scan 5. Clause structure is analysed, in terms of S, V, C etc., and the range of constructional types established. Particular care should be taken at this level, in view of its significance in so many remedial contexts (see chapter 6).

Scan 6. Phrase structure is analysed, in terms of NP, VP etc., and the range of constructions established.

Scan 7. Word-structure patterns are analysed.

Scan 8. Problem cases are scrutinized, to see if, in the light of other analyses, difficulties can be eliminated.

We incorporate three additional items of information into our analyses, solely so that our work can be more readily compared with that of other approaches: (*a*) the total number of sentences (including repetitions, but ignoring the unanalysed/problematic utterances of section A); (*b*) the mean number of sentences in each of P's interchanges with T (which we refer to as a conversational 'turn'), but ignoring turns consisting wholly of section A utterances; (*c*) an indication of sentence length measured in terms of institutionalized words, i.e. items surrounded by spaces—again, ignoring section A utterances. Statistical means are given.

(iv)　Structure count

Each instance of a structure is tabulated, and numerical scores transferred from our roughwork sheets to the Profile Chart. This chart is simply a summary of the classifications suggested on earlier pages. It contains information that is both synchronic (sections A, B, C, and the information about length) and developmental (Stages I–VII). Two instances of a completed chart are given below, one of a normal 3½-year-old, the other of a normal adult. The normal adult chart has no typological value, of course: it is a random sample of 30 minutes taken from an informal conversation about their work between two male teachers, and is therefore biased in terms of educational background and subject-matter (extracts from this data are presented in Crystal and Davy 1975, nos. 3 and 10; the profile is of speaker A). This profile shows both the strengths and weaknesses of the classification chart, when used with more mature forms of language behaviour: the basic structural features clearly emerge, as does the absence of errors in Stages VI and VII; but there is a high proportion of 'Other' constructions, showing the extent to which we have simplified the full analysis of adult language for practical purposes. These profiles are given on pp. 106–7 below.

In addition to the above general remarks, it may be helpful to explain in detail the way in which our charts are prepared, before they emerge in their final form. (We shall in fact describe what we did for one of the profiles mentioned in this book—the third profile of Mr J, the patient discussed in chapter 8.) We take as our starting point the stage where the tape has been fully transcribed, and we assume that the grammatical analysis set out in chapter 3 has been fully understood. Our main purpose here is not to illustrate the categories of the grammatical analysis that we are using, but to show how the entries thus recognized and counted are incorporated into the Profile Chart. This profile is given on p. 108.

First we prepared a worksheet, intermediate between transcription and chart, on which we made an entry for each instance of one of our descriptive categories, following the order of Scans outlined above.

Scan 1   *Unanalysed:* 6
    1 Unintelligible: 6
    2 Symbolic noise: 0
    3 Deviant: 0

    Problematic: 65
    1 Incomplete: 59
    2 Ambiguous: 6

Notes:
(*i*)   Under 'Unintelligible' we counted the following:

   1 T   goòd/
        P   (2 syllables)   *whispered*
   2 T   'what's wròng/
        P   (2 syllables)
   3 T   'what's he dòing/
        P   (syll.) the .
   4 T   same as thàt one/
        P   (2 syllables)
   5 T   'listen agàin/
             is she ríding the 'horse or/ .
        P   (syllable)
   6 T   'this one's fàt/ and 'this one's thìn/ but it 'doesn't
             'matter 'just nŏw/
        P   [snə̀us mən]/

(*ii*) Under 'Incomplete' we included any instance of sentences such as:

   1 T   'what's this 'man 'doing/
        P   ríding a/ .
   2 T   'what's this one 'then/
        P   the 'man is .
   3 T   'look at this one 'then/
             'this is thé/ .
        P   the . 'thin man .

Notice that we would not include the following under this heading:

   4 T   'who is thìs/
        P   the . fàt 'man/

since the intonation here suggests that Mr J was responding with an appropriately elliptical sentence (omitting SV in an SVC structure). Comparing *3* and *4* above should make this clear.

Scan 2   *Responses*

1 T's Questions		58	*2* T's Others		155
P's responses:					
Full major		6			38
Elliptical	1	13			24
	2	5			
	3	0			
	4	0			
Minor		12			44
Abnormal, struc.		0			0
	Ø	5			4
Repetition		8			19
Problems		0			0

Notes:

(*i*) In cases such as the following, the question of which of T's sentences to take as stimulus is resolved by the absence of pause and the asterisk convention (cf. p. 92):

T   do 'you 'know what she's sup'posed to be dòing/
P   sŏng/
T   yès/ yès/
    so 'what would she be doìng 'then/
    *do you rèad a 'song/
P   *the 'girl is .

(*ii*) Under 'Full major', we found examples such as:

T   the màn/
P   the . 'man is . 'kicking a . fòotball/

(*iii*) 'Elliptical' included the following types:

1 T   wĕll/ is the 'man púshing/ or ríding/ or drìving/
   P   drìving/   (single-element elliptical response)
2 T   the mán/ is dòing 'something to the 'football/
   P   the 'man is . kìcking/   (2-element elliptical response)

(*iv*) Under 'Minor' we recognized such cases as:

1 T   thàt's it/
   P   yès yes/
2 T   mhm̀/ wèll/ the 'apple's not 'eating the măn̆/ ìs it/
   P   nò no no/
       nò/

The sequences of *yes* and *no* were not analysed as sequences of distinct minor sentences when they lacked separate prosodic identity, e.g. we counted two minor sentences in the last contribution of Mr J here, not four. (For a discussion of Mr J's use of such sequences, see chapter 8.)

> *3* T   the 'man is 'smoking a cigarètte/
> P   yés/ — —
>   I — I — I cán't/ — —

I can't was here taken as a stereotype, hence falling within the 'Minor' category; there is a further discussion of this point below.

(*v*)   Lack of response showed up in the transcription in the following way:

> T   yès/
>   'what about one of thèse ones/ — — —
>   'what's hè doing/

It is clear that T produced the last stimulus only after no response had been forthcoming to the previous one.

(*vi*)   'Repetition' refers to repetition of T's stimulus, or a part of it, as in:

> T   'what's the gìrl 'doing/
> P   'the . 'horse is .
> T   mhm̀/ wèll/ I 'want the gîrl/
> P   'the . 'girl .
>   'the . 'girl .

Notice that the contribution from Mr J here contains not just repetition of T's stimulus, but also a self-repetition immediately after. This information is best gathered after section B of the chart has been prepared, since everything which is left over from that section (i.e. which is not to be taken as responding to T) is either an instance of self-repetition or is to be treated as novel. This left us, in this case, with the following entries on the work-sheet:

P's Spontaneous:	*1*	Repetitions	17
	2	Elliptical major (1 element)	3
	3	Others	20
Scans 3 and 4		Connectivity:	3
		1 and	2
		2 c	0
		3 s	0
		4 Other	1
		Coordination	0
		Subordination	0

Notes:

(*i*)   The two *and* constructions were found in the following stretch of dialogue:

> T   rìght/ 'let's have it agàin/
>   'can you *tèll me/

P   *'this 'man is . rùnning/ [əd] and 'this 'man is . wàlking/
T   gòod/ agaìn/
P   'this 'man is rǔnning/ and 'this 'man is wàlking/

(*ii*) Under 'Other' we catalogued one instance where the intonation suggested that some connectivity was being achieved, although no connecting element was present in the syntax:

T   so 'you lìsten/
    *I'll 'give you thīs/ .
P   *the 'man is fǎt/ the 'woman — əm — the 'man is . thìn/

Scans 5, 6 and 7. These seemed to be scans which would provide most information, and so a separate worksheet was prepared, simply to allow enough space for all the information to be set out neatly. In these scans we firstly looked for single-element sentences, and constructions involving two or more elements; subsequently we distinguished as many different types of single-element sentences as the data seemed to warrant, and entered phrase structure details of the rest. As far as single-element sentences are concerned, the worksheet finally looked like this:

Minor:	56	*Single-element major:*	
1 Social	52	*1* 'V'	16
2 Stereotypes	4	*2* 'N'	21
3 Problems	0	*3* Other	3

Note: The four instances of *I can't* we took as unanalysed wholes, on the grounds that Mr J showed no signs of being able to use the first person pronoun on its own or in other constructions at this stage, and seemed to have no other negative constructions, and no other instances of the auxiliary *can*. These sentences therefore fall under the heading 'Stereotypes'.

Two-element sentences: 26
1 SV   17
2 VO   12
3 AdjN   1

Three-element sentences: 39
1 SVC   3
2 SVO   32
3 SVA   4

Four (or more)-element sentences: 0

Once this point had been reached we were able to briefly examine the structures that we had recorded, in order to determine which of them showed phrase-level complexity at certain points in clause structure. Thus, of the 17 SV structures,

12 showed DN at phrase level for S, and 1 showed AdjN; and 13 showed Aux v for the clause-level element, V. Four were unexpanded (a point which is not marked separately on the Chart). So we entered 13 instances of Noun Phrase (NP) structure for S, and 13 instances of Verb Phrase (VP) structure for V. In addition, the 12 VO constructions yielded a further 11 instances of DN for O. These entries were made in the following way:

X + S: NP	13	
X + C/O: NP	11	
X + V: VP	13	

We were now ready to examine in detail the phrase-level composition of the constructions we had counted. Of the 13 SV types, 12 had the form DN Aux v (e.g. *the man is walking*), so we recorded the presence of 12 DN structures and 12 Aux. 1 SV type had the form AdjN Aux v (*fat man is walking*), so we recorded 1 instance of AdjN, and added a further instance of Aux to the Aux total. Then we examined the 12 instances of VO, finding 11 of the form VDN, and 1 of the form V Pron; so we added a further 11 to the DN total, and logged the single Pron. We now merely had to record the single AdjN structure, and our phrase-level analysis of two-element constructions was complete.

We then turned to three-element constructions, adding to the running totals for each phrase-level structure in exactly the same way as described above. However, it should be noted that of the 32 instances of SVO constructions, 30 showed NP structure for both S and O (23 DN and 7 DAdjN as S, 30 DN as O). We therefore logged 30 instances of XY + S: NP and XY + O: NP in respect of these, and entered DN and DAdjN figures appropriately at phrase-level. A similar procedure was followed for the 3 instances of SVC, each showing DN expansion of S, and for the 4 instances of SVA, each showing DN for S and PrDN for A. This left the 36 expanded forms of V, which were all Aux v: these were logged under the heading XY + V: VP.

We then turned to word-level analysis, where we found only two features to be taken note of: the *-ing* ending on verbs, and the 3rd singular form of the Aux and Cop (*is*). V-*ing* occurred in 17 SV structures, 12 VO structures, and 36 SVC/A structures, making a total of 65; but to this had to be added 16 instances of a V-*ing* single-element response, so a total of 81 was recorded on the worksheet. For the 3rd singular feature, we added the 3 instances of *is* as Cop in SVC structures (*the man is fat* etc.) to the total of Aux occurrences (since all were appropriately formed) yielding a total of 52.

Our analysis at this point would have been finished, if it were not for the 59 instances of Incomplete sentences recorded in Scan 1. We set these out fairly fully, as follows (for convenience, they are here listed in order of frequency in the data):

1	DN Aux.	23
2	D.	11
3	DN.	9

4	DN Aux V-*ing*.	5
5	DAdj.	4
6	DAdjN.	3
7	V-*ing* D.	2
8	DAdjN Aux V-*ing*.	1
9	DN Aux V-*ing* D.	1
		59

Note: The full-stop convention is used here to reinforce the point that these sequences are incomplete in the data, even if superficially they might be mistaken as complete (e.g. DAdjN. here is not the same as DAdjN above, of which 7 instances have been taken into account). The main evidence for incomplete status of such sequences, as already mentioned, is lack of prosodic identity. However, we feel justified in extracting from this list and entering on the chart those features of the incomplete constructions which were identifiable regardless of the incompleteness of the sequence as a whole and which were compatible with features of structure already found elsewhere in the data. They included 38 instances of DN (see Nos. 1, 3, 4 and 9 in the above listing), 4 instances of DAdjN (see 6 and 8), 30 instances of Aux (see 1, 4, 8 and 9), and so on, and it is the inclusion of these figures which enables us to arrive finally at the statistics given in the third Profile Chart of chapter 8.

The analysis was now complete, in all essential respects. However, T understandably wants to have some measure of P's progress in syntactic control, and so as a rough guide (no more than this) we make provision at the bottom of the Chart for recording the mean number of sentences per turn that P is contributing to the session, and the mean sentence length of P's productions. We calculate the first measure by dividing the total number of sentences (excluding section A utterances) by the number of stimuli provided by T. The first number is readily obtained by adding the figures under the heading *Totals* in sections B and C; the second number is the sum of all T's stimuli, as entered on the Chart to the left of *Questions* and *Others*. In the present case, this produces 165/222, yielding a mean of 0.7 sentences per turn. For the second measure, we try to avoid unnecessary identification problems by holding to the definition of a word as 'between spaces' when counting the number of items in a sentence (what we referred to above as an 'institutionalized' word). In the case of the Chart in question, we went through the list of P's complete sentences, keeping a running total of the number of words used. This amounted to 411. This number was then divided by the total number of sentences, 165, yielding a mean length of 2.5. (This figure might be compared for interest, with the total obtained for the normal adult analysed below, p. 107.)

Three further points need to be raised. (a) As already emphasized, we stress the importance of flexibility in the use of the chart. In particular, users should be ready to add further categories to it if there are grounds for thinking that these categories are likely to be useful in the case of a specific P. For example, if at Stage IV the pattern DAdjAdjN began to emerge frequently, it could be added to the Chart separately from the general category of 'Other'. In the present case, the only occasion when we felt this to be necessary was at Stage I under 'Statement'.

(b) There are no instances of structures from Stages V–VII in this profile. An indication of how these are counted has however already been given in the appropriate sections of chapter 4. (c) We would also emphasize that there are other ways of scanning the transcription than that outlined on pp. 94–8. In particular, there is something to be said for a simultaneous analysis of clause and phrase structure (Scans 5 and 6), as in certain cases it is easier to come to a decision about the grammatical structures involved if both levels are considered at the same time, e.g. whether a PrP is A, or postmodification within NP.

At present our approach is geared to the study of change in the individual (cf. p. 22), and we are therefore happy to leave our quantitative analysis as raw figures. The main indications of progress and regression are readily evident from data in this format, and we are reluctant to embark on the use of sophisticated statistical techniques which would make the procedure much more difficult to use routinely. We do of course appreciate the need to establish better presentations of the data, but do not think this will be useful until the number of linguistic variables is somewhat reduced. At the moment, we count everything, and while in principle any structure could be of diagnostic significance and a focus of remediation, it is likely that a fairly small range of patterns will emerge regularly as being particularly important. If this is so, it will be possible to take from a sample only the most salient structural characteristics, and perform statistical analyses on them which have some predictive value for groups. As we have already explained, we are not yet in a position to do this. In our Postscript, we outline the tasks that will need to be completed before this goal can be achieved. In the meantime, all figures must be seen within the perspective of the sentence total at the foot of the Chart: a total of 16 for SV has to be interpreted differently if the overall number of sentences is 50 than if it is 150.

Unanalysed | **Problematic**

1 Unintelligible **31** 2 Symbolic Noise **2** 3 Deviant | 1 Incomplete **18** 2 Ambiguous

B   **Responses**

Stimulus Type		Totals	Repet-itions	Elliptical Major				Full Major	Minor	Struc-tural	Ø	Prob-lems
				1	2	3	4					
135	Questions	**86**	**6**	**22**	**6**	**5**		**9**	**40**	**2**	**5**	**2**
68	Others	**37**		**2**	**5**	**5**		**9**	**12**	**4**		

Normal Response / Abnormal (spanning headers)

C   **Spontaneous**   **24**   **2**   **3**   Others   **21**

Sentence Type (Stage I (0;9–1;6))

Minor **52**   Social **52**   *Stereotypes*   *Problems*

Major **95**   Sentence Structure

| *Excl.* | *Comm.* | *Quest.* | *Statement* |

'V' / 'Q'   'V' **6** 'N' **11**   Other **2**   Problems

			Conn.	Clause		Phrase		Word

Stage II (1;6–2;0)

V X	Q X		SV **8**	V C/O **3**	DN	VV **2**	-ing **4**
			S C/O	A X **2**	Adj N	V part **4**	pl **7**
			Neg X	Other	NN **2**	Int X	-ed **4**
					PrN **2**	Other **2**	-en

Stage III (2;0–2;6)

V X Y / Q X Y **1** / let X Y / VS / do X Y **1**

X + S:NP **7**	X + V:VP	X + C/O:NP **2**	X + A:AP
SVC/O **7**	VC/OA **1**	D Adj N **2**	Cop **3**
SVA **4**	VO_dO_i	Adj Adj N	Aux **7**
Neg X Y	Other	Pr DN **6**	Pron **24**
		N Adj N	Other

3s **29** gen

Stage IV (2;6–3;0)

+ S / QVS / Q X Y Z

X Y + S:NP **1**	X Y + V:VP **1**	X Y + C/O:NP	X Y + A:AP **9**
SVC/OA **7**	AA X Y **3**	N Pr NP	Neg V
SVO_dO_i **1**	Other	Pr D Adj N **2**	Neg X
		c X **3**	2 Aux
		X c X **3**	Other **4**

n't **4** 'cop **3** 'aux **3**

Stage V (3;0–3;6)

how / what / tag

and **6** / c / s **7** / Other	Coord. 1 **3** 1+	Postmod. 1 clause	1+
	Subord. 1 **4** 1+ **3**		
	Clause: S	Postmod. 1+ phrase	
	Clause: C/O		
	Comparative		

-est / -er / -ly **1**

(+) | (−)

NP	*VP*	*Clause*	*NP*	*VP*	*Clause*

Stage VI (3;6–4;6)

Initiator	Complex	Passive	Pron	Adj seq	Modal	Concord
Coord		Complement	Det	N irreg	Tense	A position
					V irreg	W order
Other			Other			

Stage VII (4;6+)

Discourse | *Syntactic Comprehension*

A Connectivity	it	
Comment Clause	there	*Style*
Emphatic Order	Other	

| Total No. Sentences **147** | Mean No. Sentences Per Turn **·82** | Mean Sentence Length **3·1** |

© D. Crystal, P. Fletcher, M. Garman, 1975 University of Reading

Profile Chart: normal 3½-year-old

A

Unanalysed			Problematic		
1 Unintelligible **3**	2 Symbolic Noise	3 Deviant	1 Incomplete **36**	2 Ambiguous	

B Responses

Stimulus Type		Totals	Repet-itions	Elliptical Major 1	2	3	4	Full Major	Minor	Struc-tural	Ø	Prob-lems
17	Questions	**17**		**1**	**1**			**6**	**9**			
40	Others	**40**	**1**					**12**	**27**			

Normal Response / Abnormal headings span the central columns.

C Spontaneous **264** | **4** Others **260**

	Minor **96**			Social **96**	Stereotypes	Problems		

Stage I (0;9–1;6) Sentence Type

Major **225**			Sentence Structure				
Excl.	Comm.	Quest.	Statement				
	·V·	·Q·	·V· ·N·	Other	Problems		

Stage II (1;6–2;0)

	VX	QX	Conn.	Clause		Phrase		Word
				SV **36**	VC/O **15**	DN **69**	VV	-ing **42**
				S C/O	AX **3**	Adj N **16**	V part **41**	pl **101**
				Neg X	Other **7**	NN **3**	Int X **3**	-ed **123**
						PrN **24**	Other **42**	

Stage III (2;0–2;6)

	VXY	QXY **1**	X + S:NP **10**	X + V:VP **7**	X + C/O:NP **15**	X + A:AP		-en **24**
	let XY	VS **9**	SVC/O **98**	VC/OA **12**	D Adj N **31**	Cop **48**		3s **120**
	do XY		SVA **27**	VO_dO_i **1**	Adj Adj N	Aux **105**		gen **6**
			Neg XY	Other	Pr DN **26**	Pron **270**		n't **76**
					N Adj N **6**	Other **28**		'cop **14**

Stage IV (2;6–3;0)

	· S	QVS **1**	XY + S:NP **41**	XY + V:VP **31**	XY + C/O:NP **53**	XY + A:AP **12**		'aux
		QXYZ	SVC/OA **78**	AAXY **24**	N Pr NP **12**	Neg V **6**		-est
			SVO_dO_i **3**	Other **21**	Pr D Adj N **12**	Neg X		-er
					cX	2 Aux		-ly
					XcX **3**	Other **67**		

Stage V (3;0–3;6)

	how	tag **3**	and **14** Coord. 1 **10** 1· **8**	Postmod. 1 **22** 1· clause	
			c **4** Subord. 1 **16** 1· **18**		
			s **44** Clause: S **3**	Postmod. 1· phrase	
	what		Other Clause: C/O **21**		
			Comparative		

Stage VI (3;6–4;6)

(+)			(−)		
NP	VP	Clause	NP	VP	Clause
Initiator **14**	Complex **57**	Passive **18**	Pron	Adj seq	Modal	Concord
Coord **6**		Complement **7**	Det	N irreg	Tense	A position
					V irreg	W order
Other			Other		

Stage VII (4;6+)

Discourse				Syntactic Comprehension	
A Connectivity **12**	it **48**				
Comment Clause **60**	there **15**			Style	
Emphatic Order **16**	Other				

Total No. Sentences **321**	Mean No. Sentences Per Turn **4·2**	Mean Sentence Length **8·0**

© D. Crystal, P. Fletcher, M. Garman, 1975 University of Reading

Profile Chart: normal adult

A	**Unanalysed**						**Problematic**			
	1 Unintelligible **6**		2 Symbolic Noise		3 Deviant		1 Incomplete **59**		2 Ambiguous **6**	

<table>
<tr><td>B</td><td colspan="2">Responses</td><td></td><td></td><td colspan="5">Normal Response</td><td colspan="2">Abnormal</td><td></td></tr>
<tr><td></td><td colspan="2"></td><td></td><td></td><td colspan="4">Elliptical Major</td><td>Full</td><td></td><td>Struc-</td><td></td><td>Prob-</td></tr>
<tr><td></td><td colspan="2">Stimulus Type</td><td>Totals</td><td>Repet-
itions</td><td>1</td><td>2</td><td>3</td><td>4</td><td>Major</td><td>Minor</td><td>tural</td><td>Ø</td><td>lems</td></tr>
<tr><td></td><td>**60**</td><td>Questions</td><td>**36**</td><td>**8**</td><td>**13**</td><td>**5**</td><td></td><td></td><td>**6**</td><td>**12**</td><td></td><td>**5**</td><td></td></tr>
<tr><td></td><td>**162**</td><td>Others</td><td>**106**</td><td>**19**</td><td>**24**</td><td></td><td></td><td></td><td>**38**</td><td>**44**</td><td></td><td>**4**</td><td></td></tr>
<tr><td>C</td><td colspan="2">Spontaneous</td><td>**23**</td><td>**17**</td><td>**4**</td><td colspan="2">Others</td><td>**19**</td><td></td><td></td><td></td><td></td><td></td></tr>
</table>

	Sentence Type									
Stage I (0;9–1;6)		Minor **56**				Social **52**		Stereotypes **4**	Problems	
		Major **109**					Sentence Structure			
		Excl.	Comm.	Quest.				Statement		
			·V·	·Q·	·V· **16**	·N· **21**		Other **3**	Problems	

Stage II (1;6–2;0)			Conn.		Clause			Phrase		Word
	VX	QX		SV **17**		V C/O **12**	DN **121**		VV	
				S C/O		AX	Adj N **2**		V part	-ing **90** pl
				Neg X		Other	NN		Int X	
							PrN		Other	

Stage III (2;0–2;6)				X + S:NP **13**		X + V:VP **13**	X + C/O:NP **11**	X + A:AP		-ed
	VXY	QXY		SVC/O **35**		VC/OA	D Adj N **11**		Cop **3**	-en
	let XY	VS		SVA		VOdOi	Adj Adj N		Aux **79**	
				Neg XY		Other	Pr DN **4**		Pron **1**	3s **82**
	do XY						N Adj N		Other	gen

Stage IV (2;6–3;0)				XY + S:NP **37**		XY + V:VP **36**	XY + C/O:NP **30**	XY + A:AP **4**		n't
		+ S	QVS	SVC/OA		AAXY	N Pr NP		Neg V	'cop
			QXYZ	SVOdOi		Other	Pr D Adj N		Neg X	'aux
							cX		2 Aux	
							XcX		Other	

Stage V (3;0–3;6)				and	Coord. **1**	**1** +	Postmod. **1** clause		**1** +	-est
	how		tag	c —	Subord. **1**	**1** +				-er
				s	Clause: S		Postmod. **1** + phrase			
	what			Other	Clause: C/O					-ly
					Comparative					

Stage VI (3;6–4;6)	(+)					(−)				
	NP		VP	Clause		NP		VP	Clause	
	Initiator		Complex	Passive	Pron		Adj seq	Modal	Concord	
	Coord			Complement	Det		N irreg	Tense	A position	
								V irreg	W order	
	Other				Other					

Stage VII (4;6+)	Discourse			Syntactic Comprehension		
	A Connectivity		it			
	Comment Clause		there	Style		
	Emphatic Order		Other			

Total No. Sentences **165**	Mean No. Sentences Per Turn **0·7**	Mean Sentence Length **2·5**

© D. Crystal, P. Fletcher, M. Garman, 1975 University of Reading

Profile Chart: Mr J's third profile

6

The linguistic analysis and treatment of language disorders

Before discussing the role of LARSP in relation to pattern evaluation, remedial goals and remedial procedures—the three stages not dealt with in chapter 5—some general remarks about the relationship of linguistics to language disorders are necessary. We hope it is clear from what has been said so far that linguistics has a powerful but restricted role to play in the analysis of language disorders. It can provide a tool for analysis, and a principled procedure, but it is no panacea. It should be remembered, in this connection, that the linguist is very much in the hands of the remedial practitioner, T. In all but a few fortunate research-cum-clinical institutions, he is totally dependent on T for his data, and he must at all points liaise with T if optimum use of his skills is to be achieved. This means that one of his first tasks must inevitably be to come to terms with the views, assumptions, techniques, and above all terminology of T. We have now had an opportunity to examine the therapeutic terminology of language disorders over several years, and on the whole we find ourselves critical of it. We find it inadequate for use as a descriptive framework with which linguistic analysis can be correlated, due to its being too vague, inconsistently applied and impressionistic. We were ourselves misled for a while into thinking that categories such as 'infantile speech', 'specific language disorder', 'functional language disability', 'child aphasia', 'child dysphasia', 'delayed language development', 'minimally brain damaged', 'expressively disordered', and so on and so forth were discrete, reasonably precise categories. We have learned to know better. We no longer feel that they have even operational value for a linguistic typology, and we have ceased to work with them. We are not competent to argue for or against their value in the wider field of abnormality as a whole, but from a *linguistic* point of view, it is clear to us that some alternative classification, based on linguistic characteristics, is much needed.

Part of the underlying difficulty is an uncertainty among researchers and practitioners as to whether there is such a thing as a distinct language disorder, independent of other considerations, especially of a psychological or neurological kind. Here the views of Piaget have been particularly influential, language development being viewed as dependent on the prior development of cognitive operations (see Piaget 1970). This might well suggest a causal relationship between a language disability and some underlying cognitive deficit, and there is some evidence to suggest that linguistic symptoms we encounter may be the result of a generalized deficit in representational behaviour. Morehead's preliminary analyses (1972, 6) 'support the hypothesis of a general representational deficit in linguistically deviant children' (though unfortunately he gives no details as to what kind of children he studied apart from saying that they had 'linguistic retardation'). Morehead and Ingram's language deviant children took twice as long over symbol-matching tasks as normal children (1973), and Morehead and Johnson argue (1972, 152): 'the less advanced the child, the more necessary it is to coordinate operative knowledge with early representational knowledge such as deferred imitation, imagery and symbolic play prior to direct language training'; and they suggest that 'therapy for pre-syntactic children should begin with those aspects of representational behavior which precede language.' (See also Eisenson and Ingram 1972.) This is something which we see being done regularly in clinics and schools, in fact. However, it does not add up to a view that all language disability is merely a reflex of some other disability. Or—to put it more cautiously—there is nothing to be gained, and a great deal to be lost, by assuming that it is so, and concentrating on the assumed nonlinguistic impairment to the exclusion of linguistic considerations. There are many arguments which support this emphasis.

A rather basic point is that our knowledge of cognitive functioning is, if anything, much less certain than our knowledge of linguistic structure and use. To pass the responsibility for remediation over to a 'cognitive therapist', therefore, is unlikely to be of specific practical value other than in relation to certain very general processes. The same applies to perceptual 'explanations', (see the critique in Rees 1973). For example, Fraser and Blockley (1973) take the view that the underlying cause of language disability is a defective appreciation of relationships of space and time; and that if this is attacked and improved, language proficiency will improve as a natural consequence. While the hypothesis is not implausible, the 'comprehensive and coherent theory of perception' which they seek (40) does not exist: as they themselves say, 'We do not know enough about the normal development of perception to be able to devise a programme, let alone how it would apply in the case of the perceptually disordered child' (43). A second argument is that while in the very early stages of language development it may be difficult to disassociate linguistic from nonlinguistic deficit, as the child gets older—and certainly with the adult—a much clearer distinction emerges. There are numerous areas of linguistic structure which have but an indirect and remote relationship to cognition, e.g. concord rules, collocational rules, some word order patterns (e.g. negative placement, question inversion), and these are often areas of error. It seems to us that no amount of cognitive training is likely to improve ability in these areas, and that the case for a specifically linguistically-principled therapy remains. Moreover, as many of these patterns are acquired fairly early, quite a high proportion of children are characterized by problems that seem to be of a specifically linguistic kind. In addition, there are many Ps whose sole deficit, so far as can be established using available assessment techniques, is in language. In all other respects—auditory, motor, neurological, psychological, social, psychiatric—results are within normal limits. For such reasons, reinforced by a dominant view within human semiotic studies which sees linguistic behaviour as being of a fundamentally different kind from nonlinguistic behaviour (cf. Hockett's notion of design-features for language, and his particular focus on duality of structure (Hockett 1958, Hockett and Altmann 1968, Lyons 1973), we insist on retaining the notion of an independent language disability, which has to be assessed and remedied within a linguistic framework.

Whatever the correct position in these matters, it should be evident that progress in the understanding of linguistic deficit will only be achieved in the context of an accurate and consistent theoretical and descriptive account of language development; and in this respect, we have found many of the explanations of this deficit in psychological terms to be unsatisfactory. This claim needs detailed support, and as a case in point we cite Fraser and Blockley's study (1973) whose main hypothesis is mentioned above. We accept that if there is perceptual disability, then this must be attacked before comprehension and production of speech is likely to develop normally. But the implementation of their theory involves contradictory linguistic considerations, the status of language in their methodology is unclear, and their analysis of P's language behaviour contains misleading assumptions, when looked at from the point of view of the above chapters. Concerning their theoretical position, they claim that their work is based on a study of the literature on language over the past 200 years; but they refer only to the more speculative, philosophical writings: no technical works of contemporary linguistics are referred to at all.[1] What they produce, in fact, is an amalgam of linguistic notions from different theories and stages of development within theories, which is inevitably inconsistent. The following sentence contains at least four incompatible theoretical assumptions, for instance: 'the child has a "schema" of speech when he can transform the elliptical ungrammatical colloquial utterances of his parents into "objects of knowing", into the "kernal [sic] sentences" which obey the universal rules of language and which carry meaning' (39). On the one hand, they say their work is close to a Piagetian psycholinguistic view of language as an integral part of cognitive activity and development (52); on the other hand, their entire discussion is couched in generative linguistic terms, which are in the last resort fundamentally incompatible with a Piagetian theory (cf. Sinclair-de-Zwart's (1969) critique of Chomsky). Then within generative grammar, 1957 notions of kernel sentences are made to exist alongside 1965 notions of transformation and 1970 conceptions of deep structure in terms of generative semantics. As a result, the basic claims of their approach remain very obscure, e.g. that their programme is 'based on the theory that the remedying of the child's perceptual disorder enables him to relate the surface structure of speech to the deep structure' (27).[2] Concerning methodology, the authors of this approach provide little detail about the role of language in their work. They claim that their approach is nonverbal, that is 'we do not treat through the defective medium' (51). But the one child they give us a detailed account of, Simon, had had considerable language contact and therapy before

[1] The nearest is an extract from Chomsky's *Language and mind*, and a 1921 introductory work by Sapir.

[2] The situation is not helped by the absence of definition of two central concepts, the ' "psychic distance" from language', and the ' "mental infrastructure" of language' (11), and the standard confusion (cf. p. 5 above) between 'grammatical relationships and syntactical [sic] organization' (10–11).

their programme started, and it is left quite unclear, in the discussion of the visual and auditory sequencing tasks which constitute part of the programme, how much and what kind of language was used to him or around him in the instructions and discussion of the tasks (22–3). It seems unlikely that the programme was carried through in complete silence, and no account seems to be taken of the language contact he was receiving outside the clinic, where he was being seen for one hour each day. In this respect, attributing the improvement obtained to the perceptual hypothesis seems premature. They put the questions: 'is it reasonable that the medium of remedial education should be the one in which his disability lies? Can a disorder of language be remedied by repetitive practice in the *medium* of language?' (36), to which they clearly anticipate the answer 'No'. But a better answer is 'It depends', as the question contains an assumption which the above chapters argue is incorrect, namely that language is a single, homogeneous structure. If one takes the view that there are *levels* of syntactic structure, however, then it is perfectly feasible to concentrate on certain aspects of syntax while ignoring others, right from Stage I. We have seen children, apparently like Simon, whose progress had been slow because his therapy had concentrated on the wrong areas of syntactic structure; focussing on the neglected areas produced dramatic improvement. There is certainly some evidence in Fraser and Blockley that they have underestimated the child's linguistic ability, e.g. they say (19) 'He learned the actual action words very quickly but could not learn the structure', yet cite *girl running* as one of the utterances used, which has excellent structure at clause level; 'he had little idea of word order in sentences', but they illustrate this by *That boy sitting —is*, which is deviant in terms of verb phrase structure only; *scissors in there* is called a 'bizarre' construction (19), whereas it is an expected Stage II pattern; elliptical speech is considered ungrammatical (39, cf. p. 13 above). And once again, we are reinforced in our belief that linguistic reasoning and technique provide an indispensable element of any remedial procedure in this area.

The one thing that has hit us forcibly since we have begun to work with the language disordered is how heterogeneous a population they are. We have never found two children or adults who are the same in all salient respects. It is quite likely that the relation of cognitive to linguistic disability will be various, displaying different kinds of interaction, severity and dependence. We are therefore not in favour of any narrow attack on a disability based on a single theoretical principle. The more broadly based the attack, using a range of linguistic and cognitive strategies, the more likely we will be to hit the target. In no sense, then, do we wish to play down the importance of seeing language within a cognitive perspective, but neither do we wish to minimize the role of independent linguistic analysis and evaluation, until such time as other research shows this to be redundant. In this respect, then, there are three tasks which remain to be done, using the data of LARSP: pattern evaluation, statement of remedial goals, and statement of remedial procedures. A discussion of these constitutes the remainder of this chapter.

Patterns and goals

This is a comparative exercise, in which the pattern of syntax established in a sample is compared with other samples of P, or other Ps, and ultimately with the expected pattern (in terms of age) for normal children or the norms of the adult language. Detailed studies of the use of LARSP in this way are provided in chapters 7 and 8. Here we simply wish to point to certain patterns which have emerged sufficiently often in our work to make us suspect that they will ultimately turn out to be of typological significance. However, in interpreting a profile, the limitations of our sampling procedure (see chapter 5) should be remembered. Perhaps the most important point to bear in mind is that the positive information it contains is always more directly useful and reliable in defining a pattern than the negative (i.e. the gaps): the presence of a score is a positive indication of ability, whereas the absence of a score may mean only that the sample is biased.

Pattern 1

A profile presenting a clear case of 'pure' delayed language would be very similar to the one given at the end of chapter 5. The distribution of structures is even across the page, and the child is producing normal quantities of speech; only the age differential is out. The goal here would be to increase the frequency of structures at the next Stage of development, maintaining a balance between levels of structure. It would be hypothesized that, as a balance of structures has been obtained so far, this is likely to continue, and that unless evidence of a specific deficit emerges, all that needs to be done is to widen the range of speech situations in which P can interact and use language. Given increased motivation and opportunity, one would expect progress without structured therapy. Such profiles are not common in clinical therapy, but are more to be found in remedial education settings, where one talks more of 'disadvantaged' backgrounds. The cases of delayed language generally seen in speech therapy clinics present much less of a balanced picture (see patterns 2–6 below).

Patterns 2–6

These comprise the majority of cases, where a general sense of language delay is complicated by total gaps in structural ability. These gaps, or areas of specific weakness, characteristically appear (a) at sentence/clause level, (b) at phrase level, (c) at word level, and (d) at discourse level.

Pattern 2

This is the most common kind of delay, in our experience. Isolated words and a few phrases may be produced, but there is a lack of any coherent relationships between them, an absence of sentence patterns, and a high proportion of ambiguous cases. The disorder pattern may be more dramatic if there has been a focus on isolated words and parts of speech in previous therapy or parental interaction.

In these circumstances, there is only one initial goal, to establish a solid foundation of clause structure. This means ascertaining in the first instance whether P has the ability to use Verbs—for as we have seen (p. 44), these have a determining role in the development of clause structure—and then systematically building up clause structure patterns (see p. 121) to match the level of phrase structure complexity already achieved. Remediation continues by trying to preserve a developmental balance between clause and phrase structure levels. (Cf. Morehead 1972, who also points to the tendency for Ps to expand phrase structure before clause structure in the early stages.)

Pattern 3

This is a pattern which often develops after therapy of pattern 2, but which is also common in an initial assessment. A reasonable clause structure is established, but phrase structure is weak. There is often a one-to-one relationship between elements of clause and elements of phrase structure, e.g. *he kick ball*. Often, the only exponent of S is a pronoun. Attempts to increase the complexity of the Subject or Object Noun Phrase lead to a loss of sentence organization, e.g. *the man ball* (V being omitted), *kick big ball* (with S being lost). T's aim here must be to slowly build up phrase structure, while reinforcing the pattern of clause structure, beginning with postverbal phrases (NPs as C/O develop before NPs as S, see e.g. Ingram 1972c, 72). Difficulty in maintaining hierarchical organization has also been noticed for adults, e.g. Myerson and Goodglass (1972, 50) say there is 'a correlation between severity of aphasia and the number of specific types of distinction a patient can mark in each phrase in his base structure'.

Pattern 4

No word-level development is a pattern which would be evident only if P has generally reached Stages III or IV. Clause and phrase structure would be satisfactory, but there would be a much reduced number of inflections, and compound words would tend to be absent. The aim must be to introduce inflections systematically, and this means bearing in mind the following points.

(*a*)   Inflections group themselves into systems (singular vs. plural, present vs. past, comparative vs. superlative), and should not be introduced without making clear the overall system of which an inflection is a part. The same principle also applies to grammatical words, such as *the*, *of*, *to*, which are also often absent in this pattern, producing the familiar impression of 'telegraphic' speech. Thus, the plural *-s* must be introduced in contrast with the singular, *the* in contrast to *a* and 'zero', and so on. It is fallacious, one must remember, to conclude that the child who says *boy* for both singular and plural objects is getting the singular right and the plural wrong. On the contrary, he lacks the distinction altogether: and it is theoretically possible—though not very likely—for him to use the form *boys* to refer to both.

(*b*)   The cognitive problems posed by the various inflectional endings and grammatical words are of different kinds. Some are simply matters of concord, involving no cognitive difficulty (e.g. 3rd person singular), others are extremely problematical (e.g. comparison).

(c)   Many inflections appear in different forms, depending on the context, e.g. the allomorphs of plural, possession, past tense, etc., or the variation between -er/-est, and more/most. Presenting stable contrasts is important, particularly if P has poor phonemic discrimination.[3] (For further discussion of morphological development, see Stage II of Brown 1973.)

Pattern 5

This pattern displays strong word level development, with correspondingly weak clause and phrase structure, i.e. the reverse of pattern 4. This is a pattern which has from time to time been noticed in ESN children (e.g. Newfield and Schlanger 1968; cf. also Shriner and Miner 1968; Dever 1972b). Morehead and Ingram (1973, 342) suggest that inflections, being more evident features of surface structure are found to be easier for Ps whose general rate of learning is slow; certainly in their data the deviant group used some word structure features more frequently than the normal group (especially -s (number), -ing, contracted copula and possessive 's). In such circumstances, the aim should be to focus on clause and phrase structure, as in patterns 2 and 3.

Pattern 6

Here there is little or no recursiveness, complex sentence patterns or sentence connectivity. P may produce one-sentence utterances only, or may string a number of sentences together with little or no linguistic or logical connectivity between them. The goal here is to develop sequencing ability, using conventional story-telling resources, or games, and to promote dialogue situations, perhaps using question-response games with increasingly long sequences (simplified versions of Twenty Questions etc.).

Pattern 7

Here there is a normal distribution for age, but very few instances for a half-hour sample. There may be an abnormally high frequency of repetition. Such samples may indicate a disorder; on the other hand, they may simply reflect a sampling problem (e.g. the child being unwell during the session) or just a quiet child. A further sample should be taken, and questions of personality raised. In the extreme case, of course, the profile might be completely blank: P produced nothing, staying completely mute, or evincing only nonlinguistic vocalizations. In such

---

[3] One should note the great functional load carried by /s/ in English inflections. Articulatory difficulty here will inevitably lead to reduced morphological distinctions. It should be emphasized, however, that we are here speaking of standard English only. Many varieties of English (e.g. West Indian) do not have -s endings in some functions as a quite normal feature of their language system. For a general discussion of sociolinguistic variation of this kind, see Trudgill 1973.

cases, as we have already pointed out (p. 23), the role of a procedure using syntactic techniques is negligible, and those of the psychologist and psychiatrist must precede. The profile might be used in an indirect manner, as a means of assessing the kind of language used by T to P, and the importance of doing this should not be under-estimated. But apart from this, when faced with cases of autism, elective mutism, and the whole range of noncommunicating person, for whatever reason, the procedure advocated in this book ceases to be relevant.

Pattern 8

The main feature here is the high proportion of 'other' constructions and deviant sentences (cf. p. 28), e.g. *he want drink to, kick quickly ball man*. It is not common to find this in speech samples. It is more common in the writing samples of adult Ps. Cf. Myerson and Goodglass (1972, 44), who refer to patterns such as OV as being unlikely to be due to a wrong syntactic rule, but due to semantic salience: 'It appears likely that he strings components together in an order determined by the psychological importance of the units constituting the utterance.' In this respect, the output is similar to the constructions produced by deaf adults who are following the conventions of a signing system such as the American Sign Language.[4] With such profiles, the first thing that must be done is to investigate separately the reasons for the inflated 'other' categories, and to see if specific patterns of deviance can be detected, e.g. whether it is at phrase level, clause level, in the verb phrase only, and so on. The nondeviant pattern can be approached along the same lines as above (patterns 2–6).

Pattern 9

This profile displays a clear scatter of usage ahead of a focal point, and unexpected gaps. This is the main difference between adult and child Ps. The majority of adult sentence patterns will be in or around a given stage, but there will be sporadic strength beyond this, e.g. the bulk of the utterances may be at Stage III, but the auxiliary and modal verbs might be well preserved (Stage VI). This would be a common pattern for many Broca aphasics (cf. Myerson and Goodglass 1972, Spreen and Wachal 1973). This pattern is well illustrated in chapter 8. An additional characteristic of adult disability may be noted here: we refer to this as 'incipient structure'. This may take the form either of an unexpected breakthrough in an area that T is systematically working on, or of a sudden emergence of structures which are apparently unrelated to the current concerns of the remediation procedure. In the first case, T's attention will naturally be alerted to what is happening; and often T may justifiably conclude that simply by starting to work on a particular area of language structure contact has somehow been made with a previously 'isolated' or 'blocked' ability, and it may be possible to proceed without further delay to

[4] See Stokoe 1972, Crystal and Craig (in press). ASL and other 'natural' signing systems must be contrasted here with the 'contrived' sign systems such as the Paget-Gorman, or Seeing Essential English, which follow English morphology and syntax more exactly.

the next part of the procedure. Indeed, it may be desirable to do so, in view of the danger of over-using material with the adult patient. In the second case, however, we have problems on two accounts: it is quite possible that T, whose attention is properly focused on the task in hand (say, developing phrase structure in V forms) may fail to notice what is happening elsewhere (e.g. sudden emergence, or increase in the use of, pronoun forms for S or O), at least for some time. There is also the problem of what to do—stick by the original programme? follow the emergent structure? or attempt to compromise? An example of this difficulty is discussed in chapter 8.

With such profiles, the aim would be to consolidate and build upon the structures present at the focal stage, preserving a balance between the various levels of structure. Isolated patterns ahead of the focal stage would be temporarily ignored, but used as the starting point for therapy when the later stage was reached.

Pattern 10

This shows a full chart, with very high frequencies, a large number of stereotyped utterances and repetitions, and some low-level errors. Very fluent aphasic speech would produce this kind of pattern. It is often impossible to break into the flow or slow it down. The only alternative is to start from scratch, attempting to build up a new 'dialect', based on the developmental progression above.

Pattern 11

The profile distribution is almost identical with the normal adult one displayed in chapter 5, the only main difference being the extremely high proportion of incomplete sentences. These would have to be examined separately to determine any underlying pattern. This profile is typical of Ps with 'word-finding' problems. It is an area about which, for the moment, we have nothing to say, and for which a syntactic remediation procedure seems of little value.

Remediation procedures

Once some kind of disorder pattern has been hypothesized, the aim of the exercise is to bring P down the LARSP chart in as controlled a way as possible. Exactly how the various structures are to be introduced is the question which now has to be answered, and while the linguist may be able to offer some helpful suggestions, we would emphasize that decisions concerning the choice of remedial procedure are strictly not his to make. Deciding on the appropriateness or otherwise of a line of action we assume to be the final responsibility of T, who has to take into account such questions as motivation, availability of materials, P's general performance, etc. In this final section, therefore, we restrict ourselves to certain general guidelines concerning this boundary area between linguistics and remediation, which we have found with experience to be reasonably successful. We list them under two headings: *Positive* and *Negative*.

Positive

Faced with the problems of eliciting a structure from P, instilling some practice in its use, and planning a sequence of learning patterns, it is essential that T be aware of the many structural techniques which have been devised for these purposes, and develop an understanding of the strengths and limitations of each technique. It will not always be the case that a structural approach to therapy is what is needed, of course. Particularly with children at the very beginning of therapy, it may be inappropriate to use structural techniques for more than a small part of the time, or perhaps even not at all, until T gains P's confidence and some measure of control over his behaviour. Such decisions are not ours to make; but we do advocate that T's intuitive sense of appropriateness, timing and flexibility be supplemented by an informed awareness of what structural approaches have to offer, so that a rational decision can be made. In this, mother-tongue remediation has a great deal to learn from the field of foreign-language teaching, where studies in the use and appropriateness of structural drills have been in progress for over half a century. It is however remarkable how little the remedial language professions have been influenced by this field. We have come across few therapeutic studies which have attempted systematically to take into account the methods of structural approaches to language teaching (or more recent approaches),[5] or which have even been aware in general terms of what the foreign-language teaching (L2) methodology has to offer. Of course there are considerable differences between the two fields, which must not be underestimated. In particular, L2 drills presuppose a shared awareness of the conventions and expectations of communication (e.g. a sense of knowing when to respond) which may be quite lacking in the mother-tongue context. Also, there is a fairly widespread dislike of 'mechanical' procedures in remediation, where the basic motivation of the learner to perform willingly a structured set of tasks may be absent, and where, accordingly, T needs to approach the use of drill techniques bearing in mind the need for flexibility and moderation. Many L2 drills are more appropriate for the language laboratory situation, or for group classroom use, and it is evident that a great deal of further study of the premisses and expectations of each drill needs to be made before one can make use of them in remediation, or decide in a given instance whether the drill concept can be used at all. But it is equally evident that the L2 literature can provide an invaluable source of suggestions about the nature of language games and structural drills, and the problems of using them, as well as reminders of general language-learning principles, all of which are of potential relevance to the task of language therapy. It is for this reason that we refer now to such standard accounts as Mackey 1965 (see especially Appendices A and B) and Stack 1971 (especially chapters 7 and 8), as a perspective for evaluating the suggestions we make.

Our analyses of T–P sessions have shown that inevitably T takes the initiative in the majority of interactions, and that T's stimuli can be classified into a number of basic functional types, each of which could be the basis of structural drill.

---

[5] One exception is the use made of Hornby's structural patterns in *Guidelines* (Thomas 1971).

1   Imitation tasks. 'Elicited' or 'rote' imitation requires P to repeat the whole or part of an utterance, following an instruction such as 'Say what I say'. A sequence of imitation tasks, with increasing complexity of structure, may be introduced in this way. These tasks are currently attracting great interest in psycholinguistics, as it is thought by some that a subject's performance—in particular, the changes he introduces into a sentence he has been asked to imitate—can indicate his level of grammatical development (see, e.g. Slobin and Welsh 1968, and above, p. 86). But this conclusion is still tentative, and in remediation contexts its applicability is untested. Imitation tasks seem to be of limited value, in that without their large-scale use on a P, they can tell us very little about how far the child has used his own linguistic system to produce the sentences: he might be reconstructing it himself, as far as he is able; or he might be parrotting it.

2   Modelled imitation is much more useful as a teaching tool in remedial contexts. This is our term for the commonly-used technique of obtaining from P spontaneous utterances which follow T's model, as part of their respective roles in a highly-structured (e.g. game) situation. Examples are given throughout chapter 7.

3   Incremental drills, in L2 contexts, refer to cases where the learner is asked to complete a sentence begun by T, sometimes with a fixed phrase, sometimes with any construction. In therapeutic contexts, there is frequent use made of the 'prompt' (e.g. *It's a blue*—with expectant, rising intonation), but, as this term suggests, it is not usually used as a systematic teaching technique. We find prompts of dubious prognostic value, and of restricted use, as clearly not every part of a sentence can be readily prompted.

4   Replacement or *substitution* drills are much less commonly used in therapy than in L2 contexts, and we are unclear as to why this should be so, as they are of great potential value in remediation. These are drills in which a stimulus sentence is repeated by the learner with one or more items substituted. The teacher may provide the item to be substituted (e.g. T. *The boy was running. He.* → P. *He was running.*) or some other means may be found to motivate the substitution, such as pictures (e.g. T. *I can see a car* → P. *I can see a boat.*). A whole sequence of replacements can be made, in a 'chain' replacement drill or game, e.g. *X can Y the Z* → *X can W the Z* → *V can W the Z*, etc.

5   There are many other types of drill pattern, some of which we cite here to provide a more adequate illustration of the scope of the language teaching enterprise: none of these, however, seem to be systematically used in remediation. (The names given to each drill vary somewhat in the applied linguistic literature.)

(*a*)   Expansion drills ask the learner to add items to a stimulus sentence, e.g. T. *He comes on Mondays. Sometimes.* → P. *He sometimes comes on Mondays.*

(*b*)   Contraction drills ask the learner to shorten a sentence, such as by collapsing two sentences into one, omitting a word or phrase, or replacing a complex construction by some shorter form (e.g. a Noun Phrase by a Pronoun).

(*c*)   Embedding drills would require the learner to combine two sentences by

incorporating one within the structure of the other, e.g. T. *X is there. X is a Y.*
→ *P. X, who is a Y, is there.*

(*d*)   Transformational drills introduce structural changes into a sentence, such as
the change from active to passive, positive to negative, or changes in word order.

6   *Question-answer* drills need separate attention, as the use of a question
stimulus usually accounts for the majority of T's interaction patterns with P.
Apart from the linguistic classification of questions into structural types (see
chapter 3), T needs to be aware of the demands made upon P by the choice of
one question pattern over another. For example, it is easier to respond to
SV-inversion questions (e.g. with a nod of the head) than to Question-word
questions, which usually require some verbally specific explication. Probably the
most difficult kinds of question (or question substitute) are those which are
intended to elicit a general answer, e.g. *What's happening?*, *Tell me what he's doing*,
What can you see? These—'open-discussion' stimuli—are a very common type
of question used by Ts in the data we have analysed. Their difficulty is that they
give little or no syntactic help to P in deciding how to answer, and they may
presuppose the abilities one wants to teach (e.g. by demanding a verb in the response,
when P may not have a command of verbs—see further below), or stimulate too
wide and unconnected a range of sentence patterns in response (as is the case with
many fluent dysphasics). Handling open-discussion stimuli is we believe one of
the most advanced skills for P to learn, and he should therefore be introduced to
them with caution.

The alternative to open questions is to restrict structurally the possibilities of
response in some way, and the main technique we use here is one we refer to as
forced alternative (FA) questioning.

FA questions always conform to the basic pattern *Is it X or Y?* Their role is
to give P the linguistic stimulus required for his answer (thus minimizing nonlinguistic problems of recall, attention etc.) but without giving him a direct imitation
task. P has to choose which alternative to respond with, and in making his choice
he is forced to use his knowledge of the linguistic system. To decode an FA he has
to know it is a question and has to determine the meanings of the two alternatives.
He must then decide which of the two alternatives is appropriate for his response.
There is therefore something more than imitation involved in this type of processing.
Where the FA, as compared with a simple question, helps the child is in ensuring
that he does not have to recall from long-term memory the name of the action or
object he wants as he is processing his response (see Huttenlocher 1974, for a
discussion of the additional complexity involved in recall of object or action names
for production). If the right level of FA is selected by T, he should answer appropriately. If too advanced a level is selected, either he will not answer at all, or he
will produce a random or echolalic response. The other strength of the FA technique is that it can be focused on any part of sentence structure, and can thus be
a way of controlling P's exposure to different elements or combinations of elements.

At the risk of overemphasizing this technique at the expense of others, it may
be helpful to illustrate in detail how it is used, and to discuss some of the problems

which the introduction of a structural drill presents. (A similar level of detail would have to be considered in applying *any* of the drills mentioned above, of course.) The classical build-up of clause structure, using FA, for a child at Stage I who can name objects but do little else,[6] would proceed in six steps as follows. (We emphasize, once again, the importance of flexibility in adopting any such line of action. FA techniques, like any structural drill, can do more harm than good if used in too mechanical, rigid and unfeeling a way.)

(*i*)   *Elicit Verb* (using toys, pictures, etc. in the usual way), e.g.

> T   is the 'man rúnning/ or is the 'man sleèping/
> P   (if he is going to answer at all) rúnning/ *or* rùn/ *or* sleèping/ *or* sléep/ . . .

Notes:

(*a*)   Various possible intonations are shown. The rising and level variants may indicate uncertainty on P's part, as of course might other variations, e.g. in articulation. These problems are ignored here, and in what follows, for the sake of exposition.

(*b*)   Using the more natural elliptical patterns of adult speech (e.g. *is the man running or sleeping*) we find hinders the eliciting of the correct reponse; likewise to use pronouns (*is the man running or is he sleeping*)—presumably because these structures place too great a comprehension burden on a P at Stage I (but cf. below).

(*c*)   This pattern should be used with a wide range of Verbs, making sure that the correct reponse varies between medial and final positions in the stimulus sentence. Intonation should be kept constant (rising-type tone on the first Verb, falling-type tone on the second), except where there is a strong echolalic tendency or recency effect, in which case extra stress may be given to the first Verb, when this is the desired response. In all cases, the structure must be used, once mastered, in as wide a range of natural situations as possible.[7]

(*d*)   Correct choice of the inflection is not important at this step (as it is not, in normal development), and should not be allowed to interfere with the development of the clause structure pattern. There should certainly be no tendency to correct P's utterance unless the focus of the correction is on the structure being elicited— in this case, the Verb.

(*e*)   If P does not respond to a FA question, it may be repeated a number of times, at varying speeds and loudnesses, altering the order of the Verbs, adding cue phrases to focus attention, pointing to a sequence of pictures, or to the Verbs in their written form, if this is possible. There are no rules about this: it is up to the individual T how long he spends with a particular stimulus question before moving on. It is to be hoped that some variations in the stimulus will emerge as being more conducive to eliciting a response in P than others.

[6] If even naming is difficult, then this must first be combated; but here we find conventional therapeutic techniques to be already available. We assume that in all FA questions, comprehension of the lexical items used has already been established.

[7] Ingenious use of FA situations can sometimes be carried too far. We have heard one story (which is probably apocryphal) of a T who, when P fell off his chair and broke a leg, asked 'Is your leg broken or is your arm broken?'!

(*f*) When P responds fairly predictably, and with little hesitation, to sentences such as the above, T may move on to elicit further structures (see below). Notes (*a*)–(*e*) also apply to these subsequent steps. We can offer no guidelines as to how long it will take to get from one step to another. In some children, it has taken only 3 or 4 hours to get from here to step (*vi*) below; in others, regular sessions over a 3-month period were needed before step (*vi*) was arrived at.

(*ii*)   *Elicit O*, e.g.

    T   is the 'man 'eating an ice-créam/   or (is the 'man) 'eating a càke/
    P   ice-crèam/ . . .

Notes:

(*a*)   The ability of P to name objects is one thing; the ability to use a noun as the Object of a Verb is quite another. Before we can elicit two-element sentences of a VO type, then, we must be sure that P is aware of O as a functional element in clause structure.

(*b*)   As the structures to be elicited increase in elements, a FA question inevitably gets longer, and there may come a point where P is unable to retain the whole sentence. If T suspects this, some degrees of ellipsis may be introduced (indicated by the parenthesis in the example). This holds even more strongly for later steps, especially for longer structures after step (*vi*).

(*c*)   Verbs which have both transitive and intransitive uses make for good continuity at this step. A verb like *eat* can be used for both (*i*) and (*ii*), whereas a verb like *walk* could be used only for (*i*), and a verb like *see* could be used only for (*ii*).

(*d*)   O patterns are approached before S, for reasons already explained (see chapter 4).

(*iii*)   *Elicit VO*, e.g.

    T   is the 'man 'brushing the flóor/   or 'kicking a bàll/
    P   'brushing flòor/   *or* 'brush the flòor/ . . .

(*iv*)   *Elicit S*, e.g.

    T   is the mán 'eating/   or is the làdy 'eating/
    P   màn/   *or* màn 'eating/ . . .

Note: If P optionally produces the verb as well, this suggests T can move straight on to the next step of elicitation.

(*v*)   *Elicit SV*, e.g.

    T   is the 'man eáting/   or is the 'lady drìnking/
    P   'man eàting/   *or* 'lady drìnk/ . . .

(*vi*)   *Elicit SVO*, e.g.

    T   is the 'man 'kicking a báll/   or is the 'lady 'eating a càke/
    P   'man 'kick bàll/ . . .

This is a schematic outline of a procedure for getting from one-element to three-element structures. In real life, of course, all sorts of other factors interfere, as chapters 7 and 8 show; but in principle we think it important to keep some such progression in mind and aim towards realizing it, despite these other factors. A similar procedure could be used for eliciting multiple-element phrase structure, e.g.

T	is it a réd 'ball/ or a grèen 'ball/
P	rèd/ *or* rèd 'ball/ . . .
T	is it a 'red báll/ or a 'green èngine/
P	'green èngine/ . . .

(We have often seen this kind of elicitation being routinely used by clinicians, though not as systematically, or in as graded a way as our approach insists upon.) Once some complex phrase structures are available, an attempt can be made to get these used in clause structure. Here, though, it is important not to underestimate the difficulty of making this hierarchical 'jump', and we therefore recapitulate the above progression with a complex O, e.g.

(a)	T	is the 'boy kícking the 'ball/ or hòlding the 'ball/
(b)		is the 'boy kícking the 'big 'ball/ or hòlding the 'big 'ball/
(c)		is the 'boy 'kicking the bíg 'ball/ or 'holding the rèd 'ball/
etc.		

We have found that when structures reach this level of difficulty, it is essential for T to come to a session well prepared with a range of structures that can be realistically drawn or acted out. It is remarkable how difficult it is to think up plausible structures on the spur of the moment in the middle of a session.

Lastly, in this section, it is important to try to establish a reasonable spread of structures within a step, before moving on to the next step, e.g. questions as well as statements, phrase structure as well as clause structure—what we have referred to above as 'balance'. T should always look retrospectively at the profile classification chart, to see what gaps remain from earlier steps, and attempts to fill these should be made at the earliest possible moment. It will always remain a matter of personal decision, though, when T feels it is time to move on, or time to consolidate further, or (as was suggested above) time to stop using the structural approach for a while. Here, there is no rule of thumb. The sense of a P being 'ready' is not something which we are able or wish to make objective.

Negative

In this section we point to certain lines of action which tend to cause problems for Ts wanting to develop syntactic abilities in a structured way. It is important to emphasize, of course, that these recommendations have no necessary force in relation to other aspects of T's work, where, for example, it may be necessary to go against points 1 and 2 below in order to make any contact with P at all. Our point is simply that such variability can detract from a structured approach, once a decision has been made to try using one.

1   Not to ask P questions which presuppose the linguistic ability that it is the purpose of T to establish. If, for example, it has been shown that P is weak on clause structure, and Verbs in particular, T should avoid asking him 'open-ended' questions which would require the use of Verbs in order for any answer to be formulated, e.g. *What's the man doing?* (expected answer *Verb-ing*), or *Tell me what's happening*, which also presupposes the use of a Verb in the response. *What's that Noun used for?* is another common Verb-presupposing pattern. These questions are easy to introduce into remedial sessions, and they are frequently used; but they make grammatical assumptions which need to be carefully watched. Likewise, if one asks a question which involves three elements of clause structure in the production of the response, one is compounding the difficulty, e.g. *Why is he crying?*, *What happened next?* Questions such as this last (used e.g. by Lee and Canter 1971) should be avoided in any structural elicitation sequence, as they are too open-ended to be able to be brought under structural control: they could be answered by almost any type of sentence. Inverted questions (e.g. *is he running?*, without any alternative) should also be avoided, because of the perfectly normal tendency to monosyllabic responses, *yes, no.*

2   Not to reinforce the wrong answer. This is very easy to forget, especially with a P who has been making little progress, and where managing to get anything out of him at all is a bonus. A typical example is as follows:

T   (pointing to a picture of a man sleeping in a bed) 'what's the 'man dòing/
P   bèd/
T   yês/ that's right/ it's a bêd/ isn't it/ — it's a nîce 'bed/
      etc.

This technique, in which T takes the response obtained and builds further therapy on it, carries with it the obvious danger that T is helping P in what he can already do, and *not* focussing on the area of disability. P is avoiding the Verb in this example, and T's approach also avoids it. This is a common mistake made by parents of language-disordered children; for example, they take their child through a picture-book, naming objects, and reinforcing only the nouns which the child may come out with.

3   Not to use baby talk. But only in the sense of not using the syntactic patterns matching the child's own level. (We have no objection to the use of 'baby' vocabulary, e.g. *doggie, quacky-duck.*) Normal speech patterns should be used, though these may be of a simpler structure than in normal adult speech, as happens in normal parental interaction with their children (cf. Gleason 1973). The aim is to use structures 'slightly more advanced' than the child is using (as say Lee and Canter 1971, 318; see also Fygetakis and Ingram 1972) There is some evidence that children respond better to language levels a stage ahead of them (Shipley *et al.* 1969). Once again, these generalizations apply only to children where one is intending to try out a structured approach, and where there seems to be a reasonable chance that some progress will be made The more 'non-communicative' the child is, of course, the greater will be the tendency to use reduced forms of sentences, and in many cases, especially with subnormality, one will often have to have recourse to speaking in telegraphic form and in single-word sentences, using emphatic prosody But with such cases, the use of a structured approach is not likely to be particularly helpful. The dangers with not talking in natural syntax to a child with whom one is presenting syntactic structures in a graded way are twofold: (a) T will not speak consistently; and (b) the child will be faced with a world containing greater linguistic variety than is necessary. This happens particularly in talking to deaf children: a policy of speaking slowly and distinctly is not necessarily going to help the child to lip-read more fluently, for instance, as the majority of the situations which he will encounter will involve speech of normal speed. A child who has already made some progress in coming to grips with normal-speed lip movements might then find slow movements more difficult. The use of telegraphic speech also complicates the syntax learning process.[8] We therefore advise that when using a procedure such as LARSP the vast majority of syntactic patterns used in inter-action with P should be normal—in the sense of 'possible adult sentences'. The only slight artificiality we have introduced is in avoiding certain normal adult elliptical patterns, in the interests of preserving the parallelism of FA exercises (cf. above).

4   *Not to assume that errors always indicate disability, and need direct correction.*
It is often the case that errors can give a clear indication of where P is making progress: he is trying to use a new syntactic rule, and getting it wrong to begin with. The point has been observed for adults, too, e.g. by Sefer and Shaw (1972, 88), who see an increase in association errors as a sign that the patient's language abilities are improving (but that retrieval is defective). Nor do all errors need correction immediately. Many errors will spontaneously self-correct, if P is left to himself, and appropriate positive reinforcement given, e.g.

P   that 'man be gòing/
T   yès/ 'that's ríght/ the 'man's gòing/.

This, incidentally, seems to be the normal pattern of correction by parents, who more regularly correct in terms of the truth/falsity of a sentence, automatically introducing the proper grammar as they do so (cf. Brown and Hanlon 1970, 45–9, and also Nelson *et al.* (1973), who show that recasting of syntax in responses—that is, providing new sentences, instead of just expanding them—can facilitate acquisition (they were using a 32- to 40-month sample)). One should also note two further points in any discussion of error. (a) One should distinguish 'natural' errors from deviance: a natural error is one which is a predictable part of normal syntactic development (and to some people should not be called 'error' at all); a deviant error is one which falls quite outside the normal patterns of development of the adult language (cf. p. 28 above) . (b) The perspective of this book is standard British English. Regional dialect variation (internationally and intranationally) must be taken into account whenever it occurs. The term 'error' is out of place in any comparison of regional syntactic patterns with standard English.

---

[8] We have heard of one case where P was making no progress with normal speech, but shot ahead when T, in desperation, was reduced to talking in a telegraphic style; but unfortunately no systematic record was made, so it is difficult to be sure of what exactly happened.

5   Not to vary the stimulus sentence too much. This is particularly important with Ps with severe comprehension or attention difficulties, where a slight change in stimulus structure may be equivalent to presenting a totally different pattern. What T has to be particularly careful about here is to control the prosodic component of his speech as far as possible—keeping the intonation and rhythm constant (cf. p. 58).

6   Not to forget about pronunciation, in dealing with syntax. This may happen, for example, if one is attempting to build up inflectional endings in pattern 4 above. It is easy to overemphasize the pronunciation of the endings, so that the overall rhythm and intonation of the sentence becomes disturbed. There is nothing wrong with a clearer pronunciation of endings than normal, as long as the relative weights of these to the rest of the word and sentence are retained. In a different connection, it is important to remember always to interrelate P's phonological and syntactic abilities. If there is an articulation disorder, the emphasis we follow is not to focus on this until syntax has developed to some extent (see further chapter 7). Full pronunciation of isolated words without corresponding sentential ability can later be a hindrance in developing rhythmical connected speech, as has often been pointed out, where the individual words retain their full sound qualities and an overarticulated and arhythmic impression is the result. On the other hand, it is important not to let syntactic therapy go too far ahead of phonology: as sentences get longer and come to be used in a wider range of contexts, the possibility of ambiguity and unintelligibility due to phonological reasons increases. (This may often not be noticed by T, or P's parents, as they are used to interpreting the deviant articulation.) Regular, systematic checks on phonological development ought to be made throughout any syntactic procedure, to ascertain any general progress, to indicate any areas which may fruitfully be given immediate therapy, and to ensure that the phonological abilities which may be needed to expound a grammatical contrast are in fact present (e.g. the -*s* ending in morphology).

7   Not to try to elicit a structure without checking on comprehension first. Just as P's phonological abilities ought to be related to his syntactic, so must his semantic abilities. Our approach has been oriented towards the analysis of production (cf. p. 24). In investigating the acquisition of syntax, though, it is essential to remove interference from other linguistic levels as much as possible, and establishing semantic ability in the vocabulary used is a crucial first step. Hence, T must check that the names of all objects, events etc. are comprehended by P, e.g. by nonverbal tests, such as pointing, before a structure is introduced.

8   Not to get sidetracked. It regularly happens that, while attempting to elicit a structure X, structure Y appears. This happens particularly with adult Ps, where the attempt to 'uncover' a particular structure triggers off other structures (which are usually ·at the same stage of development—see for example chapter 8). It is inviting chaos, however, to follow up these incidental emergences in a casual way during the session in which they appear. We see a therapy session as an attempt to put into practice hypotheses about language development which have been carefully worked out in advance of the session. And the hypotheses a particular session tests are only one link in a whole chain of hypotheses which the analyst is in the process of working through. It is all too easy, we find, to become enthusiastic when an unexpected structure emerges, and to immediately spend time on it; the danger is that in retrospect it will be seen to have disturbed the general logic and ordered progress of the approach, possibly making therapy decisions about future grading of structures more difficult. As far as possible, we try to get through in a session what we plan to get through. One should always expect the unexpected —but it can be followed up next time.

9   *Not to leave too long a gap between sessions.* We do not know what the optimum amount of exposure is for syntactic remediation work, but we feel that there is little point in attempting a systematic procedure unless P can be seen for at least one hour a week, and ideally for two or three. For Ps who may be seen once a month or less, there is no point in attempting remedial procedures of the kind introduced in this book.

10 · *Not to leave too short a gap between sessions.* Obviously, there must be time left between sessions to enable the results of one's approach to be evaluated, and new hypotheses formulated. It is not necessary to do a fresh profile between each session—one every month or so might suffice, as a general check on progress. But specific decisions about the choice of structure to be introduced, consolidated or left need to be made session by session. If sessions are left to pile up without any analysis, the point of our procedure becomes lost.

11   *Not to rely too much on home practice, without prior training of the contact.* Making use of the parent or spouse of P is sometimes suggested as a way round the problems cited in 9 above. But we find that unless the kin are given careful tuition in the kind of thing T is trying to do, they can be a hindrance as much as a help. It is not easy for people with no linguistic training to appreciate the abstract nature of syntax, and the multifarious relationships between patterns that are involved. Training sounds or improving vocabulary are relatively simple tasks for family to get involved with; but syntax is very difficult. A typical error, for example, is to overdrill; to pick on a pattern, drilling it rigidly, and accepting as correct only a small range of possible responses (e.g. disallowing elliptical responses, and insisting on a 'full' sentence each time). With proper guidance, this difficulty can be removed, but it requires time and patience on T's part, and a willing and intelligent home contact, to be successful.

Many of these cautionary points, as well as the positive ones, will be illustrated by the two case studies which follow. They have been chosen from among our first attempts to use LARSP intensively, and they thus illustrate some of the unanticipated difficulties which arose, as well as the strengths of the approach. Chapter 7 applies the approach to a child; chapter 8 to an adult.[9]

[9] Cf. also the approach of Gottsleben, Tyack and Buschini (1974).

7

Case study of a child

This account concerns a boy, Hugh, who was 3;5 when therapy began. At that time he had an effective productive language capacity of single lexical items. From the beginning, LARSP was used systematically for assessment of P's progress and for structuring remediation. After four months of therapy (averaging two 45-minute sessions a week), Hugh had a well-established clause-level syntax; he was producing two- and three-element phrase-level structures, exhibiting phrasal coordination, and using a limited set of pronouns consistently. Despite a still somewhat impoverished phonology, he was conversing in a fashion much more suited to the second half of the third year of life than to the first half of the second year. This chapter presents in some detail the course of the therapy with Hugh over these months, and charts his developmental progress from Stage I to Stage IV. Syntactic profiles of the various stages are presented and analysed, and details of the remediation procedures which were attempted to advance Hugh from one stage to the next are discussed.

It will be obvious from the account below that our therapy sessions were somewhat atypical, since there was often more than one adult present. Almost all the sessions were attended by at least one of the authors, at first as an observer, and then, as time went on, as a participant in various activities. Most of the sessions were also attended by the boy's father, who played a full part in session activities. Obviously this number of adults, all able to present the relevant utterance models to the child, is not usually available to T. This does not, however, mean that the procedures we used are not possible in the normal remediation environment, with T and P only: on the contrary, most of the techniques we describe can, with appropriate modifications, be readily applied by T alone.

This case study was based on a close cooperation between T and a linguist. Each session was taperecorded. As soon as possible after each session, linguist and T discussed it, and planned structures and methods of implementing them for the next session. This kind of cooperation was essential to test the detailed applicability of our procedure, but it is perhaps worth emphasizing that it is neither necessary nor practicable when working routinely. Our approach can be applied by T working independently, once the general technique has been learnt.

Background

Hugh is the youngest of four boys, and was born at term after a normal pregnancy.

There were no abnormalities apparent in his development generally apart from the language delay. At 22 months he was admitted to hospital after a febrile convulsion which followed influenza, tonsilitis and otitis media. At 3;2 he was again admitted to hospital following a febrile convulsion, which was again associated with tonsilitis. It was soon after this that he was first referred for speech therapy. Audiological examination then indicated that his hearing was within normal limits. At the time he was first referred for therapy, he achieved the following scores on the Reynell Developmental Language Scale: Comprehension 3;9, Expression 1;6. Apart from his language, Hugh, when referred for therapy, was a normal healthy child. No other psychometric data is available for him; test situations had been avoided as far as possible because they tended to produce anxiety in the child.

The initial assessment

The major initial problem was understanding what Hugh was saying. Until some work had been done at the beginning on his phonological system, it was impossible to assess his syntactic ability. The first two therapy sessions were devoted to obtaining information about his sound system, by getting him to name items placed before him, and also by the administration of the Edinburgh Articulation Test (see Anthony *et al.* 1971). Data from these sources, and also an increase in our comprehension through familiarity enabled an accurate transcription to be made of the third session, and it was on this that the first profile was based.

Table 1 lists some of the more common substitutions made by Hugh in his utterances during the first two sessions. It might of course be argued that, since his phonology was so deviant, a systematic approach to improve his intelligibility was at least as important for his communication potential as the syntactic intervention described below. Ideally, one would like to work on phonology at the same time as syntax, particularly as phonological deficiencies can interfere with productive syntactic development (see p. 126). Hugh, for example, had at the beginning no fricatives at all. At the end of six months, this situation had not improved. Since the alveopalatal fricatives /s/ and /z/ in English carry a high functional load in English, for signalling the plural, possessive and contracted *is*, Hugh's continued inability to use fricatives was bound to affect the efficiency of his syntactic system. Our concentration on syntax, however, was imposed by Hugh's reaction to any attempt to work on his phonology. He had shown in the first session that his discrimination was good, and that he could imitate any sound produced by T in isolation. But as soon as T began to work systematically on, say a fricative-stop contrast at a particular point of articulation, Hugh flatly refused to cooperate. He was apparently aware of his deficiencies—later on, he would comment on them, saying 'I can't say that' when T required him to produce a sound (or a structure) that he could not use correctly—but he was not prepared to work at developing his sound system. This was in contrast to his attitude to the work on syntax, where he was usually, within the limits of three-year-old behaviour, ready to cooperate, and to take part in whatever activity was organized.

Table 1   Common consonantal substitutions—Stage I

	Initial	*Final*
Stops	p → b	p → b
	t → d	d → g
	k → g	k → g
	tʃ → d	tʃ → d
	dʒ → d	dʒ → d
Fricatives	f → {w, g}	v → b
		θ → d
	s → w	s → d
	h → ʔ	ʃ → d
Continuants	j → {ɲ, l}	

Once the therapist had determined what Hugh's phonemic system was (and it was a highly restricted one consonantally (as table 1 indicates), with some associated vowel distortion) it was possible to concentrate on syntax. The analysis of the third therapy session appears as profile 1, and a portion of the transcript is included below (transcript 1) to illustrate the kind of communication Hugh was having with T at this point. We will deal with the profile first.

The profile is a summary of around 250 exchanges between T and P in the course of a normal therapy session. The salient features of the session are:

(*a*)   There is a heavy dependence by T on questions to elicit language from Hugh. Over 80 per cent of all the utterances of T to which Hugh responded were questions. In general, they were questions about objects or situations in front of the child— doll's-house characters, blocks, coloured balls etc.

(*b*)   Hugh produced no response to over 25 per cent of these questions. In some cases this was because he was not paying attention, or for some other external reason. In others, the structure of the question was apparently beyond his comprehension.[1] In the first case, structural difficulties can be ruled out, and external considerations adduced, because he responds to a particular structure, for example *what is it*, appropriately at one time in the session and not at all at another. In the second case, comprehension difficulties are assumed because a particular question-type is used by T often during the session, but never gets a response. One example here is questions of the *what-doing* type. At several points, Hugh is asked *what am I doing?* or *what are you doing?* and fails to respond.

His difficulty with these structures is one we will return to later: *what-doing* questions have to be answered with a verb (cf. p. 124), and Hugh at this stage is having difficulties with verbs. Another example is in questions like *what are you sweeping?* where the question-word is the object of a transitive verb. These types of questions together produced nearly half the zero responses noted on the profile.

---

[1] Apart from the original Reynell score, which indicated in general terms that Hugh's comprehension was in advance of his production, we made no systematic investigation of the relationship between these two aspects of his language ability. Our approach was pragmatic, keeping a close watch on the structures T used, to determine how Hugh responded to them. Structures to which he consistently did not respond were not used by T for a period of time.

A	**Unanalysed**						**Problematic**			
	1 Unintelligible **35**	2 Symbolic Noise		3 Deviant			1 Incomplete		2 Ambiguous **8**	

B	**Responses**												
							Normal Response					Abnormal	
						Elliptical Major				Full		Struc-		Prob-
	Stimulus Type		Totals	Repet-itions	1	2	3	4	Major	Minor	tural	Ø	lems
	200 Questions		**117**	**2**	**48**					**69**		**51**	
	21 Others		**10**	**1**	**2**					**8**			

C	**Spontaneous**				Others	

			Minor **77**		Social **77**	Stereotypes		Problems		

Stage I (0;9-1;6) — Sentence Type

	Major **50**			Sentence Structure			
	Excl.	Comm.	Quest.	Statement			
		·V·	·Q·	·V· **5** ·N· **36**	Other **9**	Problems	

		Conn.	Clause		Phrase		Word

Stage II (1;6-2;0)

		V X	Q X		SV	V C/O	DN	VV	-ing
					S C/O	A X	Adj N	V part	
					Neg X	Other	NN	Int X	pl
							PrN	Other	-ed

Stage III (2;0-2;6)

		V X Y / let X Y / do X Y	Q X Y / VS	X + S:NP	X + V:VP	X + C/O:NP	X + A:AP	
				SVC/O	VC/OA	D Adj N	Cop	-en
				SVA	VO_dO_i	Adj Adj N	Aux	3s
				Neg X Y	Other	Pr DN	Pron **4**	gen
						N Adj N	Other	

Stage IV (2;6-3;0)

		+ S	QVS / QXYZ	XY + S:NP	XY + V:VP	XY + C/O:NP	XY + A:AP	n't
				SVC/OA	AAXY	N Pr NP	Neg V	'cop
				SVO_dO_i	Other	Pr D Adj N	Neg X	'aux
						cX	2 Aux	
						XcX	Other	

Stage V (3;0-3;6)

	how / what	tag	and / c / s / Other	Coord. 1	1 +	Postmod. 1 clause	1 +	-est
				Subord. 1	1 +			-er
				Clause: S		Postmod. 1 + phrase		
				Clause: C/O				-ly
				Comparative				

Stage VI (3;6-4;6)

(+)				(−)			
NP	VP		Clause	NP		VP	Clause
Initiator	Complex		Passive	Pron	Adj seq	Modal	Concord
Coord			Complement	Det	N irreg	Tense	A position
						V irreg	W order
Other				Other			

Stage VII (4;6+)

Discourse		Syntactic Comprehension	
A Connectivity	it		
Comment Clause	there	Style	
Emphatic Order	Other		

Total No. Sentences **127**	Mean No. Sentences Per Turn **0·54**	Mean Sentence Length **1·0**

© D. Crystal, P. Fletcher, M. Garman, 1975 University of Reading

Hugh: Profile 1

Transcript 1

	T	Hùgh/ . lòok/ . 'what's thís one/ — —	*showing toy bed*
	P	bèd/ —	
	T	'good bôy/ it's a bèd/ .	
		'what shall we 'do with the gìrl/	
		shall we 'sit her ūp/ or 'lie her dòwn/	
	P	dòwn [ɲɪ]	
	T	shall we 'make her sít/ or lìe/	
	P	dòwn/ — — —	
	T	Húgh/ —	
10	P	dòwn [ɲɪ]/ dòwn/ .	
	T	yes what's thàt for/ — —	
	P	gìrl [ɲɪ]	
	T	the gìrl/ —	
	P	*yès	
	T	*is she 'going to sít/ or lìe/ .	
	P	lìe/	
	T	hḿ/	
	P	lìe/	
	T	lìe/	
20	P	yès/ — —	
	T	thère/ . 'what a'bout gràndpa/ . I mean dàddy/	*puts doll on bed*
		is 'he 'going to sìt/ or lìe/ — —	
	P	sīt/	
	T	sìt/	
	P	yēs/ — — —	
	T	ôo/ . I've 'bent his 'legs the 'wrong wày/ (*laughs*)	
		'what's he dòing/ — —	
		he's sìtting/ .	
		'what about Mûmmy/	
30	(T)	is 'she going to sít/ or lìe/ —	
	P	sīt/ —	
	T	ḿhm/ —	
		and the bòy/ — shall we 'make hìm/ . sít/ or lìe/	
		in the *bàth/	
	P	*lìe/	
	T	lìe/	
		alrīght/	
		gōod 'boy/ — — —	
		lôok/	
40		'what's dâddy/ 'got on thère/ .	
		'can you sée/	
	P	yēs/ —	
	T	it's 'his tìe/ *ìsn't it/	
	P	*yēs/	
	T	whát is it/ —	
	P	tìe/	
	T	his tìe/ yès/	
		have yŏu got 'one/	

	P	yès/ . nǒ/	*self-correction*
50	T	nò/ — have you 'got one at hóme/	
	P	yès/ .	
	T	yěs/ *whàt/	
	P	*[bàbəɲɪʔən]/	
	T	a . bòw tíe/	
	D	nǒ/ a lìttle one/	
	T	a lìttle one/ —	
	P	ḿ/	
	T	a 'little whàt/	
	P	he 'calls èverything . 'little/ he he . de'cribed	
60		it as bàby/	
	T	m̀m/ — a lìttle 'tie/	
	P	yès/	
	T	and 'daddy's 'got a . bǐg/ — — —	
	P	*1 syll.* — — — *3 sylls.*	
	T	'what's thát/ — — —	*pointing to cooker*
		'what's thât 'Hugh/ — —	
	P	*2 sylls.* — — — *3 sylls .* — — —	
	T	'what shall we pùt in the 'oven/ — —	
		shall we 'put a cáke/ or a pìe/ — —	
70	P	pìe/ .	
	T	a pìe/	
	P	yès/ .	
	T	'who's going to màke the pie/ —	
	P	mè/ —	[mʌn]
	T	hḿ/	
	P	mè/	
	T	mùmmy/ .	
	P	nò . /mè/ .	
	T	yòu/ .	
80	P	m̀/	
	T	whó's 'going to 'make the 'pie/ .	
	P	mè/	

(c)   There is a large number of unintelligible responses from Hugh on the first profile. This is partly due to his phonological deviance, and partly our relative unfamiliarity with him at this time.

(d)   The number of minor sentence responses, always either *yes* or *no*, is also high. The phonetic realizations of these lexical items were [ɲI] and [nʌm] respectively.[2]

[2] The phonetic sequence [ɲI] also appeared as a tag on the end of identifying responses. For example, at one stage in the session this interchange occurs:

T   what's thàt one/
P   'chair [ɲI]/

The tag occurs widely in the first ten sessions and then gradually disappears. It is never clear what

As far as can be ascertained from the transcripts, Hugh's minor responses are in most cases appropriate to the context. In some cases it is impossible to tell, and in others they are definitely not appropriate, possibly signalling some comprehension difficulty. These extracts give examples of the three kinds of minor responses:

(*i*)   *appropriate*

    T   whó's 'that/ — —
         is 'that Múmmy/
    P   nò/
    T   'who ìs it / . I 'think it's bàby/

The context here reveals that Hugh responded appropriately by denying that the item was mummy. Immediately following this, however, comes an inappropriate use. T is holding a baby doll, but Hugh again uses the *no* response:

(*ii*)   *inappropriate*

    T   'who ìs it . / I 'think it's bàby/
    P   nò/

An example of a situation where it is difficult to tell whether the minor response is appropriate or not comes when Hugh is being asked whether or not he would like to do something with the doll's house:

(*iii*)   *indeterminate*

    T   'shall we 'see insíde/
    P   yès/

The object of an analysis of this kind is to ensure that P is not simply responding randomly with *yes* or *no*.

(*e*)   There are 50 single-element responses, which can be exemplified from the transcript excerpt: for example, in line 2 *bed* is an instance of 'N'; in line 31 *sit* is 'V'; there are also instances which have to be classified as 'Other', e.g.

    T   'where shall I pút it/
    P   hère/

There are in addition 4 instances of Pron, which are also entered as 'Other' at Stage I, and as 'Pron' under Stage III phrase structure.

It is on the basis of (*e*), the single-item utterances on the profile chart, that this child is said to be at Stage I. The question to be asked now is whether this is a realistic assessment, or whether the child's ability has indeed been overestimated. Could the child, in the responses we have classified under Stage I, be imitating or even merely echoing a model which the therapist has given him in stimulus sentences? As a practical concern, this is an important question to ask, since on it

---

its function is. It is almost always unstressed, and it seems inappropriate to interpret it as *yes* in the sense of a request by Hugh for confirmation of the identification made by the lexical item to which the tag is attached.

depends whether T proceeds with intervention procedures designed to implement Stage II, or whether a range of functions within Stage I are to be established first.

There are several examples in the transcript excerpt for this session of a response by Hugh which consists of an item recently produced by the therapist. In line 6, for example, and again in 16, Hugh's response consists of the final item which appears in the stimulus sentence. In 23, Hugh imitates not the final item of the stimulus but the first verb of the forced alternative (FA) question. And there are various other examples in the full text of the session which could be interpreted as imitation. There are, however, counter-examples to an imitation hypothesis, which suggest that Hugh is not using this strategy exclusively. In line 2 of transcript 1, Hugh gives an identifying response *bed* which has not previously been introduced by T. Similar examples are *girl* (12) (accompanied by the [ɲɪ] particle) and *me* (74). And in fact many of the single-element responses throughout the session are of this type. They are all, however, (in the category terms of the adult grammar) nouns or pronouns. Hugh does not produce single-element responses which are verbs (again in adult category terms) unless it has appeared previously in an utterance from the therapist. In many cases, as in 16, he produces the final item of the stimulus sentence. In other cases, as in 23, he imitates an earlier item.

In other situations in which T's question requires a verb as a response, Hugh does not give it, e.g. 27, where there is no response to *what is he doing?* As we have already mentioned, no *what-doing* question at this stage gets a response from Hugh. It is not *what-questions* in general which cause difficulty, but the spontaneous production of verbs. A longer example will show the extent of Hugh's resistance to *what-doing* questions at this time:

T   'how do 'we òpen it/ — — —
     'what are you dóing/ — — —
     'are you —
     'what are you dóing/
     you're — pùshing/ àren't you/ —
     'what are you dóing/
P   [ɲɪ]

The detailed analysis of the profile of one of T's first encounters with P yields a good deal of information. In particular, his productive capacity is limited to a single lexical item, thus entrenching him firmly at Stage I. A detailed analysis of the transcript reveals the further information that Hugh's nonrepeated single-element utterances are mainly limited to nouns. This information is relevant for the design of intervention procedures intended to implement Stage II structures, for as we have seen (chapter 6), there is no point in working on SV structures, for instance, if a child is not producing verbs at his single-item stage. The establishment of a repertoire of verbs becomes an immediately priority, and if it is considered desirable to implement Stage II structures at the same time, T can concentrate on AdjN, for example, where the verb problem does not matter. There are several other phrase-level structures listed in the profile which could be used.

Stage I to Stage II: remediation

The initial assessment is complete, the overall aims of the remediation are clear, and some specific pointers to Stage II structures have been provided by the analysis. The procedures for remediation, however, remain to be described. The profile does not tell you in what order the Stage II structures are to be presented to the child, nor does it help in deciding what input structures are most valuable in achieving the desired output from the child. A good deal of linguist–therapist cooperation in this project has concerned not only the order in which to establish structures at a particular stage, but also determining the most efficient way of supplying these structures to the child. A related point which is by no means trivial is the link between the linguistic input to the child and the situation—the toys the child was playing with when a particular structure was being worked on, for instance. Control of situational variables, the 'things talked about' in the session, which entails control of vocabulary items, was a relevant factor in the child's performance. In the early days particularly, we found that opposites such as *big* and *little*, and some primary colours, were the most successful adjectives. Nouns were not so much of a problem, provided that there were not too many of them exemplified at a time. So T found Hugh's performance on AdjN structures much better when the task he was involved in was putting coloured balls on sticks, where the adjectives and nouns are highly restricted, than it was when he was playing with the dolls' house, with all its inhabitants and furniture. The latter is potentially more interesting for the child, but the linguistic models cannot be tied so closely to it, and the visual or manipulative interest seems to interfere with linguistic concentration.

These matters—order of application of structures within a given stage, type of supplied structure and method of eliciting it, and situational variables—may well vary from P to P and from T to T. However, it is hoped that the remedial procedures described for this and subsequent stages will be widely applicable. Much more information is necessary, of course, before we can be definite about whether there is an order in which structures within a stage ought to be attacked—in other words, whether there is an internal complexity to each stage. The two main remedial methods used were structural elicitation with the forced alternative question, and modelled imitation (MI). These will be referred to frequently below, but in advance of the detailed discussion some general points can be made. With a child as young as Hugh, one of the many problems faced by T is presenting the structures aimed at in as natural and unobtrusive a way as possible. It is desirable to avoid an overstructured drilling situation in which the child mechanically repeats structures presented. We also want to keep away from the other extreme, a totally unstructured 'bathe the child in language' approach. A suitable compromise is to put the child in a position where he has the requisite structures modelled for him, and is required, by linguistic or situational convention, to produce his own approximations to these structures as a response. The planned use of the FA question (see chapter 6) played a major role in the provision of structures for Hugh early on. Questions require responses, but we found simple questions to be of no help either in modelling a structure, or in getting the child to respond. The FA question, however, as we have seen, both requires a response and provides the child with a model of the structure he is expected to produce. The following examples from the first two sessions after the profile (nos. 1 and 2 in Table 2) indicate how T presented AdjN and V structures, and elicited them from Hugh:

AdjN T   'is it a bíg 'chair/ or a lîttle 'chair/
     P   bîg 'chair/
     T   is 'this a bîg 'chair/ or a lîttle 'chair/
     P   lîttle 'chair/

V   T   Húgh/ 'are you stánding/ or sîtting/
     P   sîtting/

The usefulness of this structured elicitation is underlined by examples of simple questions and responses to them in these sessions. For the AdjN structures, T is unable to get a two-element phrase from Hugh without intermediate prompts:

     T   'what's thàt one/
     P   yèllow/
     T   yēllow —
     P   hòrse/
     T   'good bôy/

As for verbs, we have already referred to the difficulty *what-doing* questions caused. Here is another example from the same session as the FA example just given:

     T   'what's he dóing/ Hùgh/
     P   in thère/
     T   'what was he dòing/ Hùgh/
     P   in thère/
     T   'what's the 'girl dóing/ (No response from P)

It was obvious that the FA, as an eliciting structure, was having much greater success at this point than simple questions, and it seems reasonable to attribute its success to the model it gives to the child.

Modelled imitation can be illustrated from session 4, when the goal structure was NN, possessor + noun. This session involved two other adults apart from T, one being referred to as 'doctor', and these three and Hugh took part in a game. Toy animals were distributed to each participant, and T began the modelling by saying *I want Hugh's pig*. The pig changed hands, and then the next adult modelled the appropriate structure, and so on. Finally, it was Hugh's turn:

     T   'now it's Hùgh's 'turn/
     P   'doctor — hòrse/

Not a particularly exciting or ingenious game, but one that was satisfactory for its purpose. It has the essential features of all other games in which we used modelled imitation: (*a*) a previously determined structure which is used in the game by all non-P participants, or simply by T if she is the only other person, as is most commonly the case; (*b*) a game situation which forces P to produce an utterance whose syntax is as near to that of the model as he is capable of, if he wants to join in the game. Often, but not always, most of the vocabulary in model and imitation will be the same, but there will be some differences.

Table 2 presents in order the most important Stage II structures that we worked on with Hugh in the ten sessions between the first and second syntactic profiles. The table gives the structure we were aiming at, the method of introducing it, and an instance of Hugh's output. The *Notes* column gives additional information which is elaborated in the commentary. The general progression is clear enough. At first, verbs in isolation were worked on, at the same time as the first Stage II structures, AdjN. Various examples of the latter were introduced, with a restricted set of lexical items: the adjectives *big/little*, colours, and nouns like *chair*, *table* which referred either to dolls' furniture or to items in the room. The colours were initially used in collocation with the word *ball*, since the task Hugh was engaged in was to place different coloured balls on to sticks. The NN structure was represented by possessor + noun, e.g. modelled as *doctor's horse*, and reduced by Hugh to *doctor horse*. He learned this structure very quickly. It was introduced in session 4, and at the beginning of the next session, this sequence occurred:

T	Húgh/ 'what's thîs/
P	còw/
T	whôse 'cow/
P	dàddy 'cow/
T	rîght/ 'what about thís/
P	dòctor 'cow/

Table 2   Stage I to Stage II

Session	Structure	Method	Example of output	Notes
1, 2	AdjN	FA	big chair	
	V	FA	walk	
3	AdjN	MI	green ball	
	V	FA	lie	
4, 5	NN	MI	doctor horse	(*a*) intransitive verb in response to simple question
	SV	MI	—	(*b*) produces SV sequence
	PrA	FA	up there	
6	V	MI	jump	
	SV	MI	—	(*c*) imperative/progressive confusion
7, 8	SV	MI/FA	sheep running	(*d*) intransitive verb
	PrN	FA	on bed	(*e*) potential D?
9, 10	VO	FA	mending car	(*f*) transitive verb

In addition to these structures consisting of two elements of phrase structure, T was also dealing with the verb problem in the first few sessions, using FA, and getting satisfactory results. There were also single instances of V and SV responses in response to simple questions. Encouraged by Hugh's use of two-element structures, and his improvement with verbs, we decided to use MI to elicit SV structures from Hugh. We used toy animals performing actions described first of all by T and then by Hugh—*the pig is drinking the water*, for instance. When it came to Hugh's turn to describe what his animal was doing, however, there was no response. It may have been unfortunate to choose SVO structures as the model, assuming that Hugh would reduce them to SV; but even when SV structures were modelled, there was still little success, and so T moved back to phrase-level, with PrA, a preposition + adverb sequence.[3]

We surmised at this point that perhaps more attention had to be paid to single verbs in isolation before we returned to SV structures, and so in session 6 imperatives were modelled using MI. The imperative routine had T telling one of the other adults in the room to *stand, sit, walk, jump, hop, run, crawl* and (very necessary) *stop*. Hugh then took over the, for him, very enjoyable task of manipulating an adult in various postures around the room. This session worked well, and so T switched to SV again, using MI with sentences like *my pig is jumping*. When it came to Hugh's turn he did not respond. Then T saw Hugh looking at his reflection in the mirror, and improvised:

T   'that's Hùgh 'there/ —
     lóok/ —
     'can you 'see Húgh/ —
     'Hugh wàve/ — —
     Hùgh 'wave/ — —
     dàddy 'wave/ — —
     dòctor 'wave/ — —
     Hùgh 'wave/ — —
     yòu 'tell them to 'do it/

That is, T took advantage of his attention wandering to model SV structures, but this time consisting of a subject + imperative verb form. The sequence continued:

T   'tell dàddy/
P   'daddy — wàving/

Hugh attempts an SV structure, with the pause indicating some uncertainty about it, presumably due to a confusion over the difference between imperative and progressive. This is understandable since (*a*) the imperatives he was working with so successfully at the beginning of the session did not have subjects, whereas the most recent models did; and (*b*) the earlier SV structures modelled for him had -*ing* endings on the verb. The confusion continues, as Hugh continues to instruct people using the -*ing* ending on verbs:

P   yòu 'waving/
D   'miss ìs 'waving/
P   'daddy — wàving/

---

[3] One of the most important attributes that T can bring to these sessions would appear to be flexibility. This may seem paradoxical, in view of the amount of preplanning that has to go into these sessions, but structuring and a degree of flexibility are not incompatible. As soon as T realized that she was getting nowhere with a planned structure, or that P was tired, she moved on, either to another structure, or to an unstructured play session for the child.

So although this interlude demonstrates the interference problems that can arise from modelling similar but different structures within the same session, it is encouraging because, once the source of interference is identified, it is apparent that Hugh is producing an embryonic SV structure. During the next four sessions, a good deal of time was therefore devoted to two-element clause structures containing verbs. We began with SV structures with intransitive verbs (note (*d*)) like *the sheep is running*, which Hugh reduced, in his response to the FA and to MI, to *sheep running*. Only after this pattern seemed well-established did we move on again to three-element model structures, using transitive verbs (note (*f*)). Models like *is Hugh mending the car or breaking the car* were reduced to VO, *mending car*. The other structure listed in table 2 which we have not yet mentioned is PrN. Note (*e*) refers to an intrusive schwa ([ə]) which starts to appear in D, determiner, position in PrN structures:

T   'where shall we 'put múmmy/
P   'on [ə] bèd/

The item appeared in a high enough proportion of PrN structures for us to wonder whether or not it was a determiner. However, it did not appear in any other noun phrases, nor was there any other sign of three-element structures at any level, so we decided to omit it from the analysis. After the tenth session, since we had been working on two-element structures with what we felt was some success, another profile was made, again using data from the therapy session, and appears as profile 2.

Stage II

The profile is an analysis of 174 exchanges between T and Hugh. This is a smaller number than in the last session analysed, which is partly attributable to Hugh producing longer structures than he did before. This kind of variability is inevitable, though, from session to session, and it is very difficult to predict within narrow limits what the total number of utterances will be. The accompanying transcript excerpt is from the middle of the session. The main features of the profile are as follows:

(*a*)   The ratio of Other stimuli to Questions is higher in this sample than in the earlier one, approximating more closely to the distribution we would expect to find in normal adult–child interaction.
(*b*)   There is a much lower proportion of zero responses. This could be the result of two factors: first, the child's improved language ability, and second, T's careful control of the complexity of the stimulus structures she uses, after the child's early indication that he is unhappy with some question-types, for instance.
(*c*)   There is a slightly smaller proportion of Unintelligible responses. This may reflect T's increasing familiarity with the child's phonological system, rather than any improvement on his part.
(*d*)   There are very few spontaneous utterances. P is as yet not initiating

A	Unanalysed					Problematic		
	1 Unintelligible **20**	2 Symbolic Noise		3 Deviant		1 Incomplete **1**	2 Ambiguous **3**	

B Responses

				Normal Response						Abnormal			
			Repet-itions	Elliptical Major				Full Major	Minor	Struc-tural	∅	Prob-lems
Stimulus Type		Totals		1	2	3	4					
140	Questions	**112**	**1**	**33**	**18**	**2**			**45**	**8**	**13**	**6**
31	Others	**20**	**3**	**7**	**4**	**1**			**8**		**1**	

C	Spontaneous	**3**	**1**	**2**	Others	**1**

	Minor **53**			Social **53**	Stereotypes		Problems

Stage I (0;9–1;6) — Sentence Type

Major **82** — Sentence Structure

Excl.	Comm.	Quest.	Statement		
			'V' **8** 'N' **17**	Other **6**	Problems

Stage II (1;6–2;0)

			Conn.	Clause		Phrase		Word
	V X	Q X		SV **7**	V C/O **7**	DN	VV	-ing **17**
				S C/O	A X **7**	Adj N **4**	V part **4**	pl **2**
				Neg X	Other	NN	Int X	-ed
						PrN **4**	Other **8**	

Stage III (2;0–2;6)

	V X Y		X + S:NP	X + V:VP	X + C/O:NP	X + A:AP	-en
		Q X Y	SVC/O **4**	VC/OA	D Adj N	Cop	
	let X Y	VS	SVA	VO$_d$O$_i$	Adj Adj N **1**	Aux	3s
	do X Y		Neg X Y	Other	Pr DN	Pron **4**	gen
					N Adj N	Other	

Stage IV (2;6–3;0)

			XY + S:NP	XY + V:VP	XY + C/O:NP	XY + A:AP	n't
	+ S	QVS	SVC/OA	AAXY	N Pr NP	Neg V	'cop
		QXYZ	SVO$_d$O$_i$	Other	Pr D Adj N	Neg X	'aux
					cX	2 Aux	
					XcX	Other	

Stage V (3;0–3;6)

			and	Coord. 1	1 +	Postmod. 1 clause	1 +	-est
	how	tag	c	Subord. 1	1 +			-er
			s	Clause: S		Postmod. 1 + phrase		-ly
	what		Other	Clause: C/O				
				Comparative				

Stage VI (3;6–4;6)

(+)				(−)			
NP	VP		Clause	NP		VP	Clause
Initiator	Complex		Passive	Pron	Adj seq	Modal	Concord
Coord	Complement		Complement	Det	N irreg	Tense	A position
						V irreg	W order
Other				Other			

Stage VII (4;6+)

Discourse		Syntactic Comprehension	
A Connectivity	it		
Comment Clause	there	Style	
Emphatic Order	Other		

Total No. Sentences **135**	Mean No. Sentences Per Turn **·8**	Mean Sentence Length **1·3**

Hugh: Profile 2

Transcript 2

	T	Hŭgh/ — 'what does the fîre 'engine 'do/ — —
	P	[gʌ̄k]/ —
	T	'where does it gò/ — — —
		hḿ/ .
	P	*2 sylls.* — —
	T	'where does it gò/
		does it 'go to a fíre/
	P	yēs/ .
	T	'what does it dô/ when it gèts to the 'fire/
	P	làdder/ .
10	T	there's a ládder/ yès/ and 'what does the làdder 'do/
	P	'go . úp . **1 syll.* /
	T	*go . 'goes 'up yès/. and then 'when the làdder's
		'up/ 'what do the mèn 'do/ —
	P	'water . oùt/ *2 sylls.* / —
	T	they rìde in the 'fire 'engine/
	D	ǹo/ wàter/ 'comes oùt/
	T	ôh/ — —
		and 'what does the wàter 'do/ —
	P	*4 sylls.* — stòp . 'fire/
20	D	it 'stops the fìre/ —
	T	it 'stops the fìre/
	P	yès/
	T	ḿhm/ — — and 'what do the mèn 'do 'Hugh/
	P	'on 'ladder hère/
	T	'on the làdder/ —
	P	yès/
	T	'what do they dò on the 'ladder/.
	P	'go ùp/
	T	they 'go ùp/ yès/ — —
30		and . 'when . 'when they get to the tòp 'what do they
		'do/ — — —
		hḿ/ — — —
		do they 'jump ŏff/
	P	yēs/ — — nō/ — 'come dòwn/
	T	they 'come dòwn a'gain/ — be níce/ wòuldn't it/
		just 'going *'up and 'down/
	P	*bròken *2 sylls.*/ — — bròken *2 sylls.*/ *1 syll.*
		bròken/
	T	bròken/
40	P	yēs/
	T	yès/
	P	yēs/
	T	'who do you 'think brôke it/ — — —
		do you 'think Ì bróke it/
	P	nò/ *2 sylls.*
	T	whò 'broke it/ — —
		*'little . bóy/ or a 'little gìrl/

	P	*1 syll./ — — 'little *gìrl/	
	T	*a 'little gìrl 'yes/	
50		'little 'girls wòuld 'break 'things like thát/ wòuldn't they/ — —	P nods
		yès he 'says/ knòwledgeably/ (laughter) — —	
		'where's the lâdder/ —	
	P	thère/	
	T	is 'that the lădder/	high pitch range
	P	yēs/	
	T	it's 'only a lìttle 'ladder/ îsn't it/	
	P	yès/ — —	
	T	'where's the hòse/ — for the wàter/	
60	P	2 sylls. / thère/.	
	T	on thère/.	
	P	yēs/ — 2 sylls./ — —	
		2 sylls. làdder . 'come 'up 2 sylls./	
	T	the 'ladder 'comes up thére/ yéah/ —	
	P	1 syll.	
	T	'what you gòt/	
		'what are you dòing/ —	
	P	1 syll. 'water 'out hère [ɲɪ]/ 2 sylls./ —	
	T	'turning the hăndle/	
70	D	the 'water 'doesn't come 'out of thére/	
	P	1 syll.	
	T	I 'think 'that's the hòse *Húgh/	
	P	*nò/ — 3 sylls./ 2 sylls. nò/ — nò/ —	
	T	'water 'comes 'out of thère/	
	P	wàter/ 'water [ɲɪ]	
	T	ḿhm/	
	P	wàter/ — — 2 sylls. — — 3 sylls.	
	T	'where is the fìre 'engine Húgh/	
	P	'down thère/	
80	T	'down thère/	
		yès/	
		'where ìs it/	
	P	'down thére/	

conversational exchanges, or striking out on his own. The great majority of the structures analysed are responses to some stimulus from T.

(e) The number of unexpanded minor responses is still large in proportion to the whole, and the [ɲɪ] particle is still used, though less frequently than before.

(f) The non-minor responses now divide into two categories: first, the Stage I, single-item utterances; but also, outnumbering these, are Stage II structures over a fairly wide range. At clause level, there is SV, AX and VO, and at phrase level, AdjN, PrN, VPart, IntX and PrA (classified under 'Other' on the profile). These in the main reflect the structures that were introduced into the remediation during the previous ten sessions. Some examples can be seen on the transcript excerpt:

| (line) 19 | stop fire | VO | (line) 48 | little girl | AdjN |
| 28 | go up | VPart | 79 | down there | IntX |

(g)   During this session we have the first appearance of Stage III clause structures, and one three-element phrase structure. There are 4 clause structures only, and they are all SVC or SVO. The Stage III phrase structure occurs in this exchange:

T   and 'what's thís one/
P   'big — — — rèd 'ball/

The long pause presumably indicates his uncertainty about this structure, and an earlier sequence confirms that he has not mastered the internal syntax of noun phrases with more than one adjective:

T   'what's thís/ Húgh/
P   'blue bàll/ bîg/

If this is regarded as a mistake in the word order of a single-noun phrase (which could be a matter of dispute, given that there are two tone groups here) then it is one of the very few instances noted of such errors by Hugh.

(h)   Word-level development is represented at this time by -ing forms on the verbs, and by some plurals. This is entirely expected for the -ing form and the plural in terms of normal development (see chapter 3), and for the -ing form because it was so widely used in our models; but we had not systematically modelled the plural for Hugh at all. Of course, since Hugh still had no fricatives, the only way we knew he was producing plurals was when he added an extra syllable to words like horse. The usual realization for him of horse was [ʌd]. This sequence shows two instances where he adds the extra syllable:

T   will 'that box 'go in thére/
P   nò/ nò/
T   'why nót/
P   [ʌdəd] in 'there/
T   'why nót/
P   [ʌdəd] in/
T   yès/ 'there's hòrses in 'there/

It seems reasonable to assume, as T does, that he is marking a plural here, though it cannot be established at this point whether he has been using plurals systematically.

At this juncture there are two courses of action open to T, once the profile is analysed in detail. She can either take the spread and quantity of Stage II structures as sufficient, and proceed to establish Stage III structures, or she can extend the range of Stage II structures to include all those listed on the summary chart. The disadvantage of the former approach is that it runs the risk of holding back the development of certain structures which are not worked on, while advancing others, so that an imbalance develops and persists. The drawback to the other approach is that if a child is advancing quickly, and has a particular stage reasonably well established, his motivation and subsequent progress may be affected by painstakingly going through all structures at that stage. In Hugh's case, T decided to advance to Stage III structures, as he had made good progress quickly. He had begun at Stage I at the age of 3;5, roughly two years behind his peers. In terms of the profile, he had now caught up six months in about six weeks, and she did not want to lose momentum.

Stage II to Stage III

Table 3 shows the structures modelled in the ten sessions between Stage II and the next profile taken. The format is the same as for table 3, but an extra term appears in the Method column. As well as FA and MI, there is increasing use of pictures by T to stimulate Hugh's language. The use of pictures involved either T describing a series of pictures using the appropriate structure, and then having Hugh go through them again; or Hugh simply had to describe them, without prior modelling. The pictures were carefully chosen to fit with the structures being worked on. The use of pictures, in one of these ways, appears under Method as *Pics*.

Table 3   Stage II to Stage III

Session	Structure	Method	Example of output	Notes
1, 2, 3	X + O:NP	Pics	read a book	(a) omission of
	PrDN	FA/MI	in a bowl	grammatical words
	SVO	Pics	boy painting fence	
4, 5	PrDN	MI	under the box	(b) range of prepositions
	do Imp. V	MI	don't look	(c) SVO
	AdjAdjN	FA	little red bus	(d) occur later with
6, 7	VOA	FA/MI	put it in bag	simple questions
	VO$_i$O$_d$	MI	give daddy the chair	
8, 9, 10	SVO	Pics	dog hitting white ball	
	Neg XY	MI	not a pig	(e) negation problem

The first structure listed is X + O:NP, one of the early Stage III structures. The notation stands for a structure of two clause-level elements, one of which is an O; the O consists of a phrase which contains at least two elements. The example given in Table 2 is of a VO structure with the noun phrase at O consisting of a determiner plus a noun. Pictures were used to elicit this and similar structures. Hugh's performance on this structure was variable, with responses sometimes having only single-item noun phrases. Hugh often responded, when VO was the required structure, with a verb with the *-ing* ending and a single noun, for example *climbing fence*. Occasionally, he would give SVO structures when one of the pictures had been modelled using this structure, and at other times he would only respond with one element utterances, as here:

T   it's a 'boy jùmping/
P   nò/ gîrl/ 'not bòy/ gîrl/
T   it's a gîrl 'jumping/
P   nò/
T   'what îs it/ Hùgh/
P   rùnning/ rùnning/

The picture in question showed a running girl. This sequence illustrates a technique now increasingly used with both pictures and modelled imitation. T, instead of modelling a structure by describing accurately what was going on in a picture, or in the room, would instead give a false description. The intention was to provoke Hugh into correcting her, and it often worked.

We began, then, with early Stage III clause-level structures, and then attempted SVOs. Also in the first three sessions, a three-element phrase level structure was introduced, PrDN. This was the easiest of the three for Hugh—not unexpectedly, since the sole additional complexity over similar Stage II structures was the systematic use of the determiner. Soon after the structure had been modelled in the usual ways, Hugh was able to use it in response to simple questions:

T	'is she in the kítchen/
P	nò/
T	whère is she/ —
P	'in the . bèdroom/

Occasionally he was able to do this with clause-level structures as well:

T	'what's 'happening in the pîcture/ Húgh/
P	'girl — 'bouncing — bàll/

In this case T had modelled the structure not very long before. A longer sequence from this period shows how variable his control over structures can be, depending on recency of modelling and other factors:

(T has asked Hugh if he has a fish, and then asked where the fish is kept).

	T	d'you kèep him in the sínk/ —
	P	nò/
	T	in a bóttle/ —
	P	nò/
5	T	in a bòwl/ — —
	P	nò/
	T	in a tánk/ —
	P	nò/
	T	in a dràwer/ —
10	P	nò/ — —
	D	'he's in a bòwl/ on the frîdge/ îsn't he/
	P	yès/
	D	wèll then/. you 'should've sàid/ —
	P	'bowl on the frîdge/
15	A	'bowl on the frídge/
	P	yès/
	B	whére/
	P	bówl frìdge/

Even when the PrDN model is given to him here, he does not respond, but perhaps this is because of the simple question stimuli. It is only when his father (D) tells him where his goldfish is (line 11) that he gives the response, and then he omits the first Pr and D—not surprisingly, since the father's model has two PrDN structures strung together. Finally, on being asked again where the fish is, he gets quite exasperated, and the syntactic coherence of his response breaks down altogether. All grammatical words disappear (note (a)) and we are left with two nouns only. Although it is not marked here, the phrase is said with a good deal of force by Hugh, and the rising tone on *bowl* is a high rising tone; similarly, there is a high falling tone on *fridge*. So, while he can at this point in remediation deal with some three-element structures in controlled situations, he can revert very quickly to two-element sequences outside these situations. (Compare his later sequence below, where the interchange outside the structured part of the session shows a greater assurance and linguistic maturity on his part.)

We worked on PrDN at this point not simply to consolidate three-element structures, but also to broaden Hugh's productive range of prepositions (note (b)). He had been consistently making *in/on* distinctions for some time, but now the models included *under/on top of*, *behind/in front of*, and *beside*. The game session for the modelled imitation here had Hugh describing his own position in relation to a box, as it was thought that self-orientation was easier for the prepositions he found most troublesome, like *behind* and *in front of*. This seemed to be the case, and he handled the given distinctions well.

The remedial procedures described so far have applied mostly to structures under the heading of Statements (and mainly affirmative statements at that). There was little evidence, however, that Hugh was producing, spontaneously or otherwise, other sentence types, particularly imperative and question. Commands were now introduced via MI, in the course of the modelling of another structure. T had placed items in a bag like *little red bus*, *big red bus*, *little black cow*, *big brown cow*, and was modelling AdjAdjN structures. Participants were required to name the item they wanted, then reach into the bag for the item without looking into the bag. They were told either *shut your eyes* or *cover your eyes* or *don't look*, as here:

T   dòn't 'look/ Hùgh/ . tèll 'David/ . dòn't 'look/
D   'tell him 'not to lòok/ — 'don't lòok/
P   'don't lòok/

Despite being presented with two entirely different models in the previous utterance, he used the negative imperative here correctly, and continued to do so. He also used other modelled imperatives, and then, a little later, came this spontaneous example:

T   'don't lòok/. dàddy/. 'tell him 'not to lòok/
P   'don't lòok/
T   dòn't/ — Ì stopped him 'this time/
P   'put it bàck/

Other occasional spontaneous structures at this time were SVO, for example *him got gloves*. The AdjAdjN structures were easily mastered via FA, and could soon be elicited with simple questions (note (d)).

The clause-level structures attempted next were VOA and the indirect object structure, VO_iO_d. The first was elicited initially with FA, and then the range of sentences was extended using MI. The next short excerpt shows Hugh imitating a modelled structure:

T   'what do I 'do nòw/ pùt it on his héad/ tèll me/
P   'put it . on [ə] hèad/
T   'put it on dŏctor's 'head/ 'it's a very bîg 'head/

Eventually we decided not to use pronouns in models like these, and sentences like *put the chair in the tin* were preferred. There were two reasons for this. One was Hugh's incomplete pronominal system: for example, there was no recorded occurrence at this point of *they* or *them*,[4] which suggested avoiding plural pronouns, at least in O position. The second reason was some evidence of word order difficulty in relation to pronouns in O position when associated with VPart structures. There were few instances of deviant word order throughout the sessions, as we have already remarked, and the fact that pronouns in O position caused a word order problem suggested caution in using them. This sequence gives an example of deviant order:

T   d'you 'want me to 'lift you úp/
P   yès/
T   'what do you sây/
P   'lift ùp me/

The VOA elicitation was only partially successful, with highly variable performance by Hugh. This may have been due to the unnecessary complexity of the models. Instead of beginning with simple adverbs like *here*, *there* in the A position we relied on the PrDN structures already well established as As, and had models like *put the plane in the tin* reduced to *plane in* [ə] *tin* or *put in* [ə] *tin* or *put plane in*, depending on how Hugh felt. And then at times he would, in response to similar models, produce structures like *put it on your head*.

The final clause structure listed is SVO with a two-element noun phrase at O. This was attempted because SVO was a structure he was improving at, and producing spontaneously at times. This line of attack was again only partially successful, presumably because of the complex NP. We were again trying to do too much too soon, a temptation to be avoided. Pictures were used for this structure, depicting something that could be described with a complex noun phrase at O. So models included:

The boy is hitting a yellow ball.
The lady is wearing a red coat.

---

[4] An interesting sidelight on this gap in the pronoun system is one of Hugh's responses in the administration of the production section of the Northwestern Syntax Screening Test (administered routinely at this point). The item concerns the distinction between *him* and *their*. When the therapist pointed to the picture which needed the response *their wagon*, Hugh replied with *him and him wagon*. His inability to use *their* produces a circumlocution using a syntactic feature, coordination, which is somewhat in advance of his overall ability at this point.

One of Hugh's appropriate responses came in this sequence, though he used a different verb to T in his utterance:

T   yès/ a dóg/ and a whîte ball/ còme on/ 'tell me 'all
      aboùt it/ Hùgh/
P   (*3 sylls.*)
T   'tell me 'all aboùt it/
P   'dog . hîtting . 'white ball/

Finally in this series (note (*e*)) were two sessions on negation. This was an attempt to iron out a specific problem that Hugh had with negative statements. We noticed that he had three ways of negating:

(*i*) *No* as a minor response to someone else's affirmative statement, then an affirmative of his own. For example if T said *this is a red pig*, Hugh would say *no, black pig*.

(*ii*) He denies the assertion with a Stage II negative structure, e.g. *not red*.

(*iii*) The third method he had was the most complex for remediation, since it involved him repeating an assertion, while at the same time shaking his head. An example of this appears on transcript 3, lines 42–53. Hugh is talking about the propellors on a plane in a picture. At line 43 he says *me got them*, but what follows indicates that he is denying that his jet has any propellers, and the transcription comments indicate that he was shaking his head when saying this. Since T is concentrating on his spoken output, she misses the headshaking cue, and the father notices it and brings it to her attention (line 54).

The game T devised to try to cut out Hugh's dependence on the third method was ingenious. Participants were blindfolded when it was their turn to select items out of a bag and identify them using the model *it's an X*. Others then used the model *it's not an X* when someone deliberately identified an item wrongly. Hugh was encouraged to take a major part in telling the person he or she was wrong. The blindfold ensured that headshaking would not be a useful cue for Hugh to use in these circumstances, and he consistently used the *not an X* negation form in this session. It took some time, however, before the headshaking disappeared altogether.

Stage III

The next session was analysed to assess progress towards the aim of establishing Stage III structures, and is summarized on profile 3. We shall not discuss this profile in detail, as most of the information it contains is a straightforward development of the tendencies already noted at earlier stages. It is evident that the advance through the stages is being maintained. In addition to a very small number of zero responses, less unintelligible responses, and the first appearance on a profile of spontaneous utterances, the number of Stage III structures is in advance of Stage II structures, and there is a wide coverage. There are one or two unexpected Stage IV structures, represented entirely at phrase level by structures

Transcript 3

	T	what's the làdy 'doing/ —	*pictures from*
	P	[kʌg]/ gìrl/ — slèeping/	*Edinburgh*
	T	it's a lit/ it's a gìrl/ ís it/ —	*Articulation Test*
	P	slèeping/ .	
	T	'what's she dòing/	
	P	slèeping/ .	
	T	slèeping/ — — —	
		'what are thòse/ —	
	P	'on a bìrd/	
10	T	yès/	
		they're 'on a bìrd/	
		it's 'what the 'bird flìes 'with/	
		'what do we càll them/ — —	
	P	fèather/	
	T	wìngs/ .	
		yès/	*said to herself,*
			rapid, quiet
	P	*wīng/	
	D	*fèathers/	
	T	fèathers/	
20		'what has your âeroplane 'got/	
		'not 'only the bìrds have gót them/ but your	
		aêroplane's 'got 'two of thóse/ hàsn't it/	
	P	yés/	
	T	'what áre they/	
	P	wìng/	
	T	yès/ —	
		'makes it gò 'faster/	
	P	hōuse/ — càr 'park/	
	T	a gàrage/ *or a càr 'park/	
30	P	*gàrage/	
	D	he said a *càr 'park/	
	P	*càr 'park/ he said a hùt/ a càr 'park/	
	T	yès/	
	P	*1 syll.*	
	T	it . it's nòt/ . well you do 'park the 'car in thére/	
		but it's it's a 'special 'kind of hòuse/ — and you	
		'could get pètrol 'there/	
		whàt's it 'called/ the — —	
	P	a . càr 'park/	
40	T	nó/ it's nòt the cár 'park/ the — gàrage/	
	P	gàrage/—	
		twò/ gàrage/ 'are òpen/	
		'me 'got — thĕm/ — — —	*shakes head*
		'me 'got thém/ .	*shakes head*
	T	'you've got thóse/ — m̀hm/ —	
	F	have 'you got thèse Húgh/	

P	nò/	
T	nò/. he's al'ready tòld us/ 'it's a *jét/	
P	*got thĕm/	shakes head
50 T	'those are propèllers/	
P	2 sylls./ pèller/ — —	
	'got thèm/ —	shakes head
T	you hàven't 'got them/	
D	nò/ . he's still 'shaking his hèad/	
P	1 syll.	
	. . .	
T	and what èlse did we 'have/	
P	thrèe 'christmas 'tree/	
D	thrèe 'christmas 'trees/	
P	yēs/	
60 T	what èlse did we 'have/ — —	
P	'paper — —	
T	ḿ/	
P	chàin/ —	
T	pàper 'chains/ —	
P	'paper cháin/	
T	and 'where did you 'have the pàper 'chains/ .	
	did you 'have them on the flŏor/ — —	
P	yès/ —	
T	did you 'say you tròd over them/ 'on the	
70	'paper trái/ the cháins/ — —	
D	nò/ we 'didn't have 'paper 'chains on the	
	flóor/ 'where did we hàng the 'paper 'chains/	
P	'on the/ — 'on the . chrìstmas 'tree/	
D	òh 'no/ 'not on the chrìstmas 'tree we didn't/ — —	
	'what a'bout the 'decoràtions/ 'where did we	
	'put the 'decoràtions/ — — —	
P	er — — 2 syll. / — in the . 2 syll./	
T	*on the lănding/	
D	*nò/ — we 'put them on the cèiling/ dìdn't we/ —	
80 P	'put them . in the cèiling/	
D	and 'where did we 'put the ballòons/ —	
P	on cèiling/	
D	*2 sylls.	
T	*who 'blew the bal'loons úp/ — —	
P	mé/	
D	díd you/	
P	yès/	
F	did you . did you 'blow the bal'loons ùp 'Hugh/	
	or 'did you bùrst them/ —	
90 P	'blow 'them ùp/	
F	dìd you/ 'good bòy/	

A	**Unanalysed**				**Problematic**		
	1 Unintelligible **13**	2 Symbolic Noise		3 Deviant	1 Incomplete **9**	2 Ambiguous	

B Responses

Stimulus Type		Totals	Repet-itions	Normal Response						Abnormal			Prob-lems
				Elliptical Major				Full Major	Minor	Struc-tural	Ø		
				1	2	3	4						
110	Questions	**93**	6	17	21	6			46		3	3
22	Others	**14**	4	5					6			3

C Spontaneous **2** | Others **2**

Sentence Type		Minor **52**			Social **52**	Stereotypes	Problems

Stage I (0;9–1;6)

Major **57** — Sentence Structure

Excl.	Comm.	Quest.	Statement			
	'V'	'Q'	'V' **5** 'N' **15**	Other **5**	Problems	

Stage II (1;6–2;0)

	Conn.	Clause		Phrase		Word
VX	QX	SV **2**	VC/O **2**	DN **1**	VV	-ing **10**
		S C/O **3**	AX **2**	Adj N **6**	V part **2**	pl
		Neg X **3**	Other	NN **3**	Int X	
				PrN	Other	

Stage III (2;0–2;6)

		X + S:NP	X + V:VP **3**	X + C/O:NP **3**	X + A:AP	-ed
VXY	QXY	SVC/O **6**	VC/OA **1**	D Adj N	Cop **3**	-en
let XY	VS	SVA	VO$_d$O$_i$ **1**	Adj Adj N **2**	Aux **2**	3s
do XY		Neg XY **2**	Other	Pr DN **2**	Pron **2**	gen
				N Adj N **5**	Other	

Stage IV (2;6–3;0)

		XY + S:NP	XY + V:VP	XY + C/O:NP	XY + A:AP	n't **1**
+ S	QVS	SVC/OA	AAXY	N Pr NP	Neg V	'cop
	QXYZ	SVO$_d$O$_i$	Other	Pr D Adj N	Neg X	'aux
				cX	2 Aux	
				XcX **1**	Other	

Stage V (3;0–3;6)

how	tag	and	Coord. 1	1 +	Postmod. 1 clause	1 +	-est
		c	Subord. 1	1 +			-er
		s	Clause: S		Postmod. 1 + phrase		
what		Other	Clause: C/O				-ly
			Comparative				

Stage VI (3;6–4;6)

(+)			(−)		
NP	VP	Clause	NP	VP	Clause
Initiator	Complex	Passive	Pron	Adj seq	Modal	Concord
Coord		Complement	Det	N irreg	Tense	A position
					V irreg	W order
Other			Other		

Stage VII (4;6+)

Discourse		Syntactic Comprehension	
A Connectivity	it		
Comment Clause	there	Style	
Emphatic Order	Other		

Total No. Sentences **109**	Mean No. Sentences Per Turn **·83**	Mean Sentence Length **1·6**

Hugh: Profile 3

containing *and*; coordination had not been explicitly modelled to Hugh between Stages II and III.

There are some examples of Stage III structures on transcript 3. At line 9 is *on a bird*, PrDN. There is an SVO structure at 43, *me got them*, and at line 80, a VOA *put them in the ceiling*, with an appropriate use of a third person plural pronoun (there is a model for this utterance on the preceding line, however). Line 57 has *three christmas trees*, an AdjAdjN structure. All of these had been part of the remediation procedure. There were two instances in the session of Neg XY, some instances of *no* plus explanatory assertion, and one instance (in transcript 3) of the perseverance of Hugh's headshaking negation. There were three instances of the copula *is* in SVC structures. Both examples of Aux are *can't*—presumably learned as a single item, and not a contraction of *can* + *not*, as there are neither instances of *can* nor instances of contraction in the session or indeed in previous sessions. This is one of the instances of *can't*:

T   'have you 'drawn a 'picture of your búggy/
P   nò/ . 'can't 'draw my bùggy/

Towards Stage IV

Because of the representation of SVO structures in the sample for profile 3, and its non-elicited occurrence in earlier sessions, it was thought to be the best starting-point for expansion towards Stage IV. The first sessions (see Table 4) were concerned with expanding noun phrases in S and O positions in SVO structures: this is what is indicated by XY + S:NP and XY + C/O:NP. At Stage IV, they refer to any three-element clause structure with a noun phrase in either subject or object/complement position. The model structures were of the type *the big horse is jumping the fence*, for XY + S:NP, and for XY + O:NP, *the horse is eating green grass*. We began by building up to the first model in stages—*the horse is jumping*, *the big horse is jumping*, because we knew that Hugh was variably imitating auxiliaries, and that he reduced structures too long for him rather unpredictably. This excerpt shows him with the shortest structure, *the horse is jumping*:

T   the 'horse . ís/ — —
P   jùmping/
T   yès/ yòu 'say it/
P   jùmping/
T   nò/ 'say the 'whole thîng/
P   'whole thîng/ — — 'horse is jùmping/

Apart from Hugh's little joke of literal repetition, it seems that the only item in this sequence he has difficulty with is the determiner. The next sequence, from the same session, comes when T increases the number of items in the model by adding an adjective in the NP:

T   the 'big horse is jùmping/ 'you can say thàt one for me/
P   nô/

```
T    yès/ gò on/
P    'can't sày it/
D    you càn 'say it/
T    you càn/
P    okày/
T    'go òn/
P    'horse . 'is — — jùmping/
T    gòod boy/ the 'horse is jùmping/ the bîg 'horse is 'jumping/
P    bîg horse 'jumping/
```

As soon as another item is added, Hugh cuts out one of the items he is already producing, usually the auxiliary. The only way T could get him to include the auxiliary was to shift the tonic onto it, and then Hugh would omit the adjective from the noun phrase. This trade-off strategy to solve the length/complexity problem that was troubling him was also used for the expanded O structures. It is interesting to see Hugh's own reaction to the model given him, in the excerpt quoted. He was obviously well aware of the problem on a conscious level. (We could have used the simple present tense form in the models, instead of the present progressive—*the big horse eats the grass*, for example—and so avoided the length problem, or at least alleviated it. This could, however, have caused other difficulties, cf. chapter 1.)

Table 4   Stage III towards Stage IV

Session	Structure	Method	Example of output	Notes
1, 2, 3	XY + S:NP	MI	big horse jumping	(a) influence of tonic syllable
	XY + C/O:NP	MI	pig eating the cake	(b) assurance in spontaneous exchanges
4, 5, 6	negation	MI	daddy isn't horrid	
	questions	Pics	what boy doing	
7, 8	copula	MI	polar bear is furry	(c) range of adjectives

Apart from what seemed to be only the partial success of our structured approach towards Stage IV, there were some encouraging signs elsewhere. The first spontaneous Stage IV negative structure appeared, with a noun phrase in O position: *me not like that pig*. And Hugh was showing a new assurance in nonstructured exchanges with T (note (b)).

```
T    you've 'cut your êye/ háven't you/
P    nò/ 'cut my hèad/
T    you 'cut your héad/
P    mm̀/
T    whère did you do thát/
P    'fell on the gròund/
T    did 'somebody púsh you/ or did you just 'fall òver/
P    'somebody . pùsh me/
```

There seems to be much less dependence on models for control of structure, and spontaneous utterances are more similar to structures being elicited than formerly;

e.g. *'me gòt no 'cowboy*, which is a spontaneous utterance from one of these sessions, is an XY + O:NP structure.

The next sessions, 4, 5 and 6, were devoted to the elicitation of negatives and questions. Negatives had consistently been a problem area, but there had recently been hopeful signs of improvement. Questions, in any form, had however been in short supply in Hugh's output, and if they did appear, were generally only intonationally marked. One obvious reason for this is the nature of the therapy situation. The child in therapy becomes quickly used to answering questions—we have only to look back on the profiles in this chapter to see how important questions are as stimuli—and is rarely in a position where he can learn to ask questions himself. Consequently, when he has advanced to the point where he does have conversations, he rarely asks any questions himself. As parents and teachers of preschool children will be aware, this is somewhat unusual. Another possible factor in Hugh's lack of questions may be the syntactic complexity involved, particularly with the *yes/no* questions such as *is the cow jumping*, which require subject-auxiliary inversion. Earlier, Hugh had not mastered the auxiliary, so it was not too surprising that he did not produce questions of this type. He had however, during the first three sessions after profile 3, had auxiliaries modelled for him, though not as a primary aim of the remediation, and consequently both *yes/no* questions and *wh-* questions were included in the procedures for the next two sessions.

For negation, the structures modelled were SVC of the type 'X is adj', where the adjective was inappropriate, and participants denied the assertion in their responses. After the models had been used successfully, simple questions elicited the same response. A variety of adjectives was introduced, for the ancillary purpose of widening Hugh's vocabulary range in this category; the following exchanges illustrate method and results:

T   is dóctor 'horrid/
P   nò/
T   'what d'you sây/
P   'doctor îsn't 'horrid/
     . . .
T   'daddy is a mònkey/
P   nò/ 'daddy nòt a 'monkey/
T   'daddy ísn't a 'monkey/
P   'daddy ìsn't a 'monkey/

The first sequence is straightforward. The second reveals Hugh's performance as variable, omitting an auxiliary which is unstressed in the first model, but including it when a stressed auxiliary is supplied.

The procedure for questions used pictures of children performing different actions. T modelled a question which Hugh had to (*a*) answer, and (*b*) imitate in asking T about the next picture. The question might be appropriate or not to the picture, so that negatives could be practised as well, as in this exchange:

T   'is the 'boy júmping/
P   nò/ 'boy îsn't 'jumping/

Most successful in the first session devoted to questions were immediate imitations, as in these examples for a *yes/no* and a *wh-* question:

T   àsk her/ 'is the 'boy júmping/
P   'is 'boy júmping/
. . .
T   just àsk/ 'what's the 'boy dòing/
P   'what 'boy dòing/

In the next session, Hugh managed the *yes/no* questions with a wider range of verbs. An attempt was also made in this session to get Hugh to produce fricatives, as he was still pronouncing *is* as [ɪd], for example. But these attempts were strongly resisted by the child, and, after some fruitless effort, dropped.

The final sessions in this series were given over to the copula. SVC structures containing a wide range of adjectives were introduced, to determine whether the copula could be used by Hugh with any less variability than the auxiliary *is*. Models were of the form *the animal is Adj—the tiger is stripey, the polar bear is furry, the lion is fierce*—and Hugh was more competent with this structure than with the auxiliary + *-ing* form. Any comparison, though, is vitiated rather by the difference in length between the two kinds of models.

After eight sessions a further session was analysed and summarized on the profile classification chart. This was intended as a guide for future remediation, as we were at this point unsure about Hugh's progress. We had begun by modelling early Stage IV structures like X + S:NP, had advanced to Stage IV negation and question-types with partial success, and had seen evidence of Hugh's spontaneous (or, at least, non-elicited) production of other Stage IV structures—coordination, Neg X and NPrN. At the same time, his performance on some Stage III structures, notably Aux and Cop, was variable. The summary appears as profile 4, and a transcript excerpt is included also.

The profile captures a further steady progression down the page, well into Stage IV. The early structures, which we had worked on in some detail, were well represented. Neither the Stage IV questions, nor the negatives, however, appear at all. The most interesting feature of the analysis of sentence structure is the widespread appearance of phrasal coordination (see lines 45, 70, 72 of transcript) which is something that Hugh has picked up without it being specifically modelled. This is true also for the modal *can* in line 65, and the AdjAdjAdjN structure *ten red racing cars* (line 84). In addition the adjective *same*, realized phonetically as [lam] by Hugh, had not been introduced into the session dealing with adjectives. Those sessions had left their mark, however, since the examples in the transcript show that he is using *same* as an adjective like *furry* or *stripey* in an SVC structure, describing an attribute of an individual noun rather than comparing two nouns:

P   [ən] lórry 'same/ and [ən] ràcing . car . 'same/.[5]

---

[5] We were unable to determine a consistent interpretation for the phonetic sequence [ən], which sometimes seemed to be *that*, at other times simply *the*.

Transcript 4

	T	thìs spéedboat/ is blàck/	*slow delivery*
	P	yèah/ —	
	T	dàddy/ ís 'this 'speedboat 'black/	
	D	nó/ .	
		'this 'speedbloat 'speedboat ìsn't 'black/ *(laughs)*	
	P	yĕs/	
	T	no that's bròwn Húgh/	
	P	òh/ . bròwn/ — bròwn/ bròwn/ —	
		òh/ 'motorboat . 'go hère/	
10	T	'that 'motorboat 'goes thère/ .	*rapidly*
		the ràcing-cár/ is rèd/ —	*slow delivery*
	P	nò/ grèen/ —	
	T	gò on/	
		'tell 'Doctor Flètcher/	
	P	[ə́ŋ] 'green/ and [ə̀ŋ] 'green/ —	
	T	'tell 'Doctor 'Fletcher about thìs one/	
	P	[ə́ŋ] sàme/ — ís/. thé/ sàme/ .	*same = [lam]*
		[əŋ] lórry 'same/ and [əŋ] ràcing . 'car 'same/.	
	T	ḿ/ — — — 'what's [làm] 'Hugh/	
20	D	the sàme/ —	
	P	sàme/	
	T	oh the sàme/	
	P	yès/ gréen/. ánd/. grèen/	
	T	yès/ the 'same còlour/ —	
		now lòok/	
		thòse 'two/ are the 'same cârs/ àren't they/	
	P	m̀m/ *1 syll.* ràcing 'car/ — —	
	T	thìs 'car . the sáme 'Hugh/ — — —	*slowly*
	P	yès/	
30	T	it's the 'same . cŏlour/ ísn't it/	
	P	yès/ — sáme/ . cólour/ . ís/ . thé/ . lòrry/	
	T	the 'same 'colour às the 'lorry/	
	P	ḿ/	
	T	yès/	
	P	'two mòtor 'boat/	
	T	twò 'motor boats/ alríght/ .	
		are thèy the 'same cólour/	
	P	er nò/	
	T	'what are thèy/	
40	P	réd/ —	
	T	'they're . dìfferent/ àren't they/ —	
		dìfferent 'colours/	
	P	m̃/ —	
	T	Hùgh/ are 'those càrs . the 'same cárs/ —	
	P	gréen 'one/ and a rèd 'one/	
	T	yès/ . and Hùgh/ lòok/ — 'this is 'a	
	P	*(laughs)*	
	T	Hŭgh/ — lòok/	
		'let's 'look at thèse 'two for a mínute/	

50 P   *2 sylls.*
    T   'this is a ràcing cár/
    P   ḿ/
    T   and 'this is a . tàxi . *'car/
    P   *yès/ . m̀/
    T   'so they're . dìfferent/ âren't they/
    P   'two ràcing 'car/
    T   'two ràcing 'cars/   *excited*
    P   'two mòtor 'boat/
    T   'two mòtorboats/ yès/ .
60   are 'these — the 'same cŏlour/ — — —
           'what have 'you dòne/ — —
           you've dròpped it/
           thàt's 'what 'you've dóne/ —
    P   càn/ wòrk/ .
    T   Hŭgh/
    P   'can wôrk/ — — càn/ wòrk/
    D   'yes it càn 'work/ . now lìsten/ 'let's 'play
           thìs 'game 'first/
    T   are 'these 'cars — the 'same cŏlour/ —   *slowly*
70 P   nò/ . 'yellow and — grèen/ (*laughs*)
    T   'what's thàt/ —
    P   gréen 'car/ ánd a/ — 'green . lòrry/
    T   a gréen/ cár/ and a gréen lòrry/ alríght/ —
    P   '[ən] 'go hère/ — — — 'put 'them 'like thàt/ —
    D   you 'put them like thàt/
    T   'what còlour's 'that 'saw Húgh/
    P   mè 'want/ a rèd/ 'red ràcing 'car/ . red —
    T   you 'want a 'red ràcing 'car/ —
    P   mm̀/ — —
80 T   do you 'think I've gòt a 'red *ràcing 'car/
    P   *yès/ — hère/ nò/ — yès/ — — —
    T   thàt rácing 'car/ is rèd/   *slowly*
    P   yès/ — 'got . tèn 'red 'racing 'car 'in hére/
    T   tĕn 'red 'racing 'cars in 'there/ I 'don't
           'think I hăve/ —
           shall we 'see how 'many I hàve gót/ — —
    P   'one thère/ and 'one thère/ — —   *rapidly, slurred*
           [ən] lànd'rover/ [əd]
    T   hḿ/
90 P   [ən] làndrover/ 'got a 'landrover hère/
    T   yés/ you've 'got a lāndrover/ but that's nŏt/
           1 syll. nō/ we're 'looking for 'red ràcing 'cars/
           áren't we/
    P   *1 syll./* [ʌnt] 'red 'racing/ — —
           òne/
    T   'don't think there are 'any 'more 'red ràcing
           'cars Húgh/ . I think 'that's the lòt/ —
    P   *2 sylls./* 'get 'out — nów/ — 'get 'out

A **Unanalysed**   **Problematic**

1 Unintelligible **5**   2 Symbolic Noise **8**   3 Deviant | 1 Incomplete **2**   2 Ambiguous

B **Responses**

Stimulus Type	Totals	Repet-itions	Elliptical Major 1	2	3	4	Full Major	Minor	Struc-tural	Ø	Prob-lems
103 Questions	**87**	**6**	**21**	**14**	**13**			**30**	**3**		**6**
47 Others	**41**	**1**	**10**	**6**	**5**			**20**			

Normal Response spans columns Repetitions / Elliptical Major (1-4) / Full Major / Minor; Abnormal spans Structural / Ø.

C **Spontaneous** **12** | **1** | **2** Others | **10**

Sentence Type	Minor **50**		Social **50**	Stereotypes	Problems

Stage I (0;9–1;6)

	Major **90**		Sentence Structure
	Excl.	Comm.	Quest.	Statement
		·V·	·Q·	·V· **10** ·N· **10** Other **10** Problems

Stage II (1;6–2;0)

	Conn.	Clause		Phrase		Word
		V X	Q X	SV **2**	V C/O **3**	DN	VV **1**	-ing
				S C/O **2**	A X **3**	Adj N **17**	V part **5**	**15**
				Neg X	Other **4**	NN **3**	Int X	pl
						PrN **5**	Other **2**	**2**
								-ed

Stage III (2;0–2;6)

	VXY	X + S:NP **2**	X + V:VP **2**	X + C/O:NP **2**	X + A:AP	
	QXY	SVC/O **5**	VC/OA **3**	D Adj N **9**	Cop **4**	-en
	let XY VS	SVA **1**	VO$_d$O$_i$	Adj Adj N **2**	Aux **2**	3s
	do XY	Neg XY **3**	Other **3**	Pr DN **5**	Pron **6**	
				N Adj N	Other **2**	gen

Stage IV (2;6–3;0)

	+ S	XY + S:NP **5**	XY + V:VP **1**	XY + C/O:NP **6**	XY + A:AP **1**	n't
	QVS	SVC/OA **2**	AAXY	N Pr NP	Neg V	·cop
	QXYZ	SVO$_d$O$_i$	Other	Pr D Adj N	Neg X	·aux
				cX **2**	2 Aux	
				XcX **4**	Other **2**	

Stage V (3;0–3;6)

		and	Coord. **1**	1 +	Postmod. **1** clause	1 +	-est
	how	c	Subord. **1**	1 +			-er
		tag s	Clause: S		Postmod. **1** + phrase		
	what	Other	Clause: C/O				-ly
			Comparative				

(+)		(−)	
NP	VP	Clause	NP	VP	Clause
Initiator	Complex	Passive	Pron	Adj seq	Modal	Concord
Coord		Complement	Det	N irreg	Tense	A position
					V irreg	W order

Stage VI (3;6–4;6)

Other | Other

Stage VII (4;6+)

Discourse		Syntactic Comprehension
A Connectivity	it	
Comment Clause	there	Style
Emphatic Order	Other	

Total No. Sentences **140**	Mean No. Sentences Per Turn **·96**	Mean Sentence Length **1·9**

Hugh: Profile 4

There is a sharp increase in the number of spontaneous utterances in this session, and no zero responses at all. The proportion of Other stimuli is much higher too. Minor sentences are still well-represented.

Summary

Therapy for Hugh began when he was 3;5 and had an effective productive capacity of single lexical items. When profile 4 was taken, Hugh was 3;9. Four months of remediation structured in terms of normal language development had taken him from the kind of language normally used by children eighteen months old and younger, to that more usual from two-and-a-half year olds. This chronological normalizing is of course an important aspect of language remediation for the preschool child, particularly in view of the natural parental anxiety that any language problems should as nearly as possible be removed before the child enters school. But as important as catching up in the sense that one might say that Hugh has caught up a year in four months, according to the LARSP, is the kind of improvement that is made. To move from lexical items to a point at which the main features of clause syntax have been established is a major achievement. And in addition, it seems from the evidence available that Hugh has now started to acquire language on his own, although this is not yet systematic enough for him to be left to his own devices without therapy. However, we do not yet know whether this is a general feature of this kind of remediation with a significant proportion of language-delayed children—the information is not yet available. Nor do we know, if it is a general feature, whether there is a particular stage at which it occurs. But in the case of Hugh, the emergence of this range of spontaneous language development has been an encouraging sign.

8

Case study of an adult

Introduction

In this chapter we shall try to illustrate the ways in which our procedures for assessment and remediation have been applied in the case of an adult dysphasic. We are very conscious of the fact that adult dysphasics differ very widely in both the severity and nature of their language disorder, and we realize that concentrating, as we shall in this chapter, on just one patient inevitably restricts the scope of our illustration in a rather idiosyncratic fashion. However, it should be remembered that our main purpose here is illustration, not at all a general study of adult dysphasia (which would be beyond the scope of this book), and that representativeness would still elude us even with descriptions of, say, three or four different types of patient. For the moment, we are at the beginning of things, and lack a systematic typology for what we intuitively feel to be different sorts of adult dysphasia. As we have pointed out (chapter 2), we hope that our work will eventually provide a basis for such a typology, in the field of grammar. However, all we require just now of our procedure is that it prove adequate for adaptation to individual cases, so that eventually we shall be in a position to compare certain different types of disorder within a coherent framework.

It may be that, in one or two places in this chapter, we have gone into some possibly alarming detail. We have some misgivings that some readers will be put off by this, and assume that our suggestions only lead to further complications, and pointless theorizing, in a job which is already difficult enough! Our reason, however, in each case was that we felt bound to be as *explicit* as possible. Where we took a particular decision, we wanted to set it out in such a way that the arguments, and the underlying assumptions, behind it could be examined, as fairly as possible. Quite possibly some of these arguments and assumptions are not as good as they should be; so they are opened to inspection here. Certainly, our theorizing was not pointless, since it guided our practice; our proper (and much more serious) concern now is to assess the credentials of the theorizing in this light. Most of the close discussion concerns the description of the first syntactic profile and certain points of detail that arose in the remediation procedure; we hope that the information supplied in such passages will be treated as supplementary rather than as compulsory, especially on a first reading.

We may close this introductory section with a few observations about the therapy situation as it applied in the case of the patient whom we shall call Mr. J.

The general pattern was as follows: T saw Mr J once a week, each session being fully taperecorded and subsequently followed up, a few days later, by a discussion of the tape between T and ourselves. In this way, we were able to monitor Mr J's linguistic progress; additionally, T had final responsibility for relating the linguistic remediation procedure to other factors (such as health, disposition, family situation etc.). For the first 3 sessions, T saw Mr J as an outpatient, alone; later, she saw him at home (except for 3 semi-sessions in the hospital ward, when he was an inpatient, undergoing a haemorrhoids operation). Seeing him at home made it possible for sessions to vary a good deal in length, depending on Mr J's receptivity (sometimes taking up most of a morning). His wife was also naturally involved in such sessions, and was most willing and able to cooperate with T, particularly in the matter of helping Mr J retain the work done in one session to the next.

General and medical background

Mr J was born in December 1926, and at the time of his stroke was a warehouse general manager, married, with two daughters aged 10 and 4 years. In July 1971 while on holiday in France he collapsed at a friend's house, and was admitted to Lille City Hospital. His symptoms were reported as: right hemiplegia, right homonymous hemianopia and total aphasia. No predisposing cause was found. The EEG showed a slow dysrhythmia on the left hemisphere; the angiogram showed a complete occlusion of the left internal carotid artery 1 cm above the carotid bifurcation. At first it was feared that he would not survive, or, if he did, that he would remain beyond reach of intensive rehabilitation. But, in August he was transferred to a hospital in Reading, and a rehabilitation programme was put into effect—consisting of remedial gymnastics, physiotherapy, occupational therapy and speech therapy. In October he was discharged home, it having been decided that no surgery was possible. He continued to receive all three therapies as an outpatient. He was then able to walk unaided, with a stick, but had very little use of his right arm, and was unable to work. During this time we, as linguists, were not involved. As far as his language was concerned, considerable spontaneous improvement seems to have taken place in the first half of 1972, although it is undoubtedly the case that he benefited greatly from speech therapy at that time. The therapy commenced by working on phonation and the imitation of sounds, concentrating on lip and tongue movements. (For further details concerning Mr J's linguistic ability at this time, see Child 1972.) As his comprehension gradually improved, he went through a period of depression and frustration which caused additional problems, as also his unwillingness to attempt speech for fear of making mistakes. Many areas were worked on, in the light of results obtained from the Minnesota Test for Differential Diagnosis of Aphasia (see Schuell 1965), such as reading aloud, auditory memory and sequencing, word-finding, questions and answers etc. However, the main difficulty, noted time and again, was his inability to retain work between sessions. His first speech therapist left the hospital in January 1973, resulting in further depression; and unfortunately, there was another break in therapy when his second speech therapist also left, at the end of the following summer. The present speech therapist started work with him in September 1973, and her preliminary assessment of his linguistic ability at that stage was as follows:

Comprehension: still considerable difficulty; simple commands had to be repeated.
Speech: only single words for the most part; severe word-finding difficulty; some persistent articulatory problems.
Reading: inidividual letters were distinguishable, but he was not able to read and understand a sentence; written material could, however, be used as a cue to word-finding.
Writing: able to write a few words (with left, non-preferred, hand only).

The first syntactic profile

This was established on the basis of a general elicitation session on 25 September 1973. T was newly assigned to Mr J, and wanted to discover as precisely and comprehensively as possible the extent of the language control that he had. The session was fully taperecorded, and a half-hour sample was extracted from it and transcribed for the purpose of the type of analysis set out in chapter 5. T was using throughout the session a combination of pictures (from magazines, for the most part, especially colourful full-page advertisements) and questions about the pictures—trying to allow enough time between questions for spontaneous speech to be produced, without letting gaps of silence become uncomfortably long.

We shall spend some time discussing the main features of this profile, as it differs, inevitably, in many respects from what one would expect from work with a child (chapter 7). The total number of sentences in the sample was 243,[1] with a further 52 utterances entered under category A: of these, 17 were 'unintelligible' (consisting of an undecipherable noise, usually of one syllable, or, quite frequently, an alveolar click); 30 were 'incomplete' (e.g. *'box . syll.* probably for *boxing,* where 'syll.' simply indicated a monosyllabic undecipherable sequence); and 5 were 'ambiguous' (e.g. *bòy* in response to *what's he dòing*). This leaves us with 243 sentences that we could straightaway analyse exhaustively and a further 35 which might yield to analysis subsequently. However, first we noted, in category B, how many of these 243 sentences came as *responses* to what T said (rather than as spontaneous, initiating productions on the part of the patient). We found in all just 61 responses to the questions of T and we were able to categorize them as follows: 61 normal, 7 abnormal, with 7 repetitions. Under 'normal' we recognized 5 full major types (e.g. *the boy is sìtting/*) where there is a well-formed syntactic pattern (albeit with hesitant intonation) in an appropriate response, with no ellipsis; 19 elliptical types (with either one or two elements present, e.g. *grèen/, pūl'ling 'it*); and 37 minor sentences (mainly involving *yes* or *no*—we shall return to this type presently). In the abnormal category we found 7 instances where no

---

[1] This is a rather higher figure for a half-hour sample than that obtained for profiles 2 and 3 (127 and 165 sentences respectively); see pp. 174, 175). It may fairly be considered abnormally high for Mr J., and the very high proportion of minor sentence types seems to provide the explanation. This feature of the data is discussed further on pp. 164–5.

A — Unanalysed / Problematic

A	Unanalysed			Problematic	
	1 Unintelligible **17**	2 Symbolic Noise	3 Deviant	1 Incomplete **30**	2 Ambiguous **5**

B — Responses

				Normal Response							Abnormal		
					Elliptical Major				Full			Struc-		Prob-
Stimulus Type		Totals	Repet-itions	1	2	3	4	Major	Minor	tural	Ø	lems
81	Questions	**61**	**7**	**17**	**2**			**5**	**37**		**7**	
219	Others	**170**	**16**	**33**				**9**	**128**		**11**	

C — Spontaneous

C	Spontaneous	**12**	**10**	**12**	Others

Stage I (0;9–1;6)

Sentence Type	Minor **165**		Social **165**	Stereotypes	Problems

Major **78** — Sentence Structure

Excl.	Comm.	Quest.	Statement			
	·V·	·Q·	·V· **8** ·N· **42**	Other **1**	Problems	

Stage II (1;6–2;0)

			Conn.	Clause		Phrase		Word
	VX	QX		SV **12**	VC/O **2**	DN **16**	VV	-ing **24**
				S C/O	AX	Adj N **2**	V part **2**	pl **8**
				Neg X	Other	NN **1**	Int X **1**	-ed **4**
						PrN **1**	Other	

Stage III (2;0–2;6)

	VXY		X + S:NP **11**	X + V:VP **13**	X + C/O:NP	X + A:AP	-en
		QXY	SVC/O **2**	VC/OA	D Adj N **1**	Cop	
	let XY	VS	SVA	VO_dO_i	Adj Adj N	Aux **14**	3s **14**
			Neg XY	Other	Pr DN	Pron **1**	
	do XY				N Adj N	Other	gen

Stage IV (2;6–3;0)

			XY + S:NP	XY + V:VP	XY + C/O:NP	XY + A:AP	n't
	+ S	QVS	SVC/OA	AAXY	N Pr NP	Neg V	
		QXYZ	SVO_dO_i	Other	Pr D Adj N	Neg X	'cop
					cX **1**	2 Aux	
					XcX **2**	Other	'aux

Stage V (3;0–3;6)

	how		and	Coord. **1**	1 +	Postmod. **1** clause	1 +	-est
		tag	c	Subord. **1**	1 +			
			s	Clause: S		Postmod. **1** + phrase		-er
	what		Other	Clause: C/O				
				Comparative				-ly

Stage VI (3;6–4;6)

(+)				(−)			
NP	VP		Clause	NP		VP	Clause
Initiator	Complex		Passive	Pron	Adj seq	Modal	Concord
Coord			Complement	Det	N irreg	Tense	A position
						V irreg	W order
Other				Other			

Stage VII (4;6+)

Discourse		Syntactic Comprehension
A Connectivity	it	
Comment Clause	there	Style
Emphatic Order	Other	

Total No. Sentences	**243**	Mean No. Sentences Per Turn	**0.8**	Mean Sentence Length	**1:2**

Mr J: Profile 1

response was forthcoming in a situation where one was clearly to be expected. (It should be pointed out, however, that this was never the result of uncooperativeness on Mr J's part—he was in all cases simply blocking, and a number of the unintelligible utterances came from this sort of situation, where Mr J clearly recognized that he was to speak, and was trying to do something about it.) In the 'repetitions' category we put such instances as *peóple/* (in response to *what about the peóple/*); notice the rising intonation pattern, presumably carried over, together with the word itself, from T's question.

We should note here that we found 61 to be a surprisingly low figure for category B (responses to T's questions). When we examined T's side of the dialogue, however, we immediately found the reason; there were only 81 questions in the half-hour sample. For the rest, T had used 29 commands (*tèll me/*; *trỳ it/*), 121 statements (*I don't think it's a strĭng/*) and 69 gap-fillers of various sorts (*mhm*; *yès*; *OǨ*)—that is, 219 non-questions. To these Mr J had provided 170 responses (with 11 further instances of zero-responding). Interestingly enough, the distinction in T's language between 'Questions' and 'Others' seems not to have played a role in determining the nature of Mr J's responses; the ratio of 81 questions to 219 non-questions closely corresponds to that of 61 (responses to questions) to 170 (responses to non-questions), indicating that non-questions were just as fruitful in eliciting responses as were questions. Similarly, an analysis of the sentence types shown in the responses to questions and to non-questions reveals no significant differences.

As a case in point, we may here conveniently take up the discussion of the minor sentence pattern, briefly alluded to above. The first thing to notice is the very high proportion of minor to full and elliptical major sentence types in category B (165 to 66). Great weight was being placed on the minor type, which is represented almost exclusively in the data by *yes* and *no*, in various combinations. Mr J frequently used both *yes* and *no*, in reduplicated sentences (*ah yès yes yes yes yes/yès yes yes yes/*; *nò no no no/*), apparently for the purpose of providing a well-known segmental vehicle over which prosodic contours might be established (indicating agreement, exasperation, acknowledgement and so on): we shall symbolize these repeated sequences as Yes^r and No^r. *Yes* and *no* were also used singly, for affirmation and denial; *no* frequently occurred when Mr J recognized that what he had said was wrong (often *no* in such instances formed part of the overall prosodic pattern of the utterance), though he was generally unable to correct himself. We found that the relative frequencies of these 4 types of minor sentence were as follows:

	Category B	Overall
Yes	16	90
Yes^r	9	33
No	7	23
No^r	5	19
	37	165

From this it will be readily seen that the frequency pattern in category B (responses to T's questions) is not essentially different from the overall pattern. We may conclude, therefore, that as far as the most frequently occurring sentence types are concerned, it does not really matter whether T attempted to elicit speech by asking questions or by some other means. And we suspect also that the rather low proportion of questions to commands, statements and gap-fillers on the part of T is by no means unusual (especially in work with adult dysphasics, perhaps).

Now we come to category C, which records the number and type of the spontaneous utterances of Mr J. It will be seen that these formed but a tiny proportion of the total (12/295), smaller even than that of category A. Moreover, of these 12 utterances, nearly half (5) were repetitions of some spontaneous production (i.e. self-repetitions on the part of Mr J). For the rest, we had the following novel (nonrepeated spontaneous) sentences:

1	'too ? 'false	? 'force
2	'little gírl/	
3	gòod/	
4	'twenty-six	
5	'thirty	
6	'man	
7	?'two . 'young	? too
8	'race . results	

Of these, the first represented a problem in identification—Mr J was looking at a picture of Muhammed Ali, and apparently trying hard to say something about boxing—perhaps that he felt championship fights were rigged beforehand? or that boxing is too violent? Item 7 also represented a problem, in that it was unclear whether Mr J was saying *two young* (AdjAdj) or *too young* (IntX); this was therefore counted as ambiguous. The remaining items were all analysed as elliptical 1-element sentences at clause level, in the usual way (*race results* being logged also as NN in phrase structure). The uncertain intonation of items 4–6 and the pause in item 8 we ascribed to Mr J's general lack of confidence in expression during this session, and accordingly did not treat these sentences as incomplete.

Finally, there is the stages analysis to which we subjected the utterances we were able to analyse. Under the heading 'sentence type', we recorded 165 minor sentences and 78 major, in all. These totals, of course, included the 33 instances of repetitions that had been logged already in sections B (7 + 16 = 23) and C (10). This told us at once that 33/244, or 13.5 per cent, of the utterances subjected to stages-analysis were not novel. In this case, 13.5 per cent was an acceptably low figure, so we were able to take the stages-analysis pretty much at face value. Notice that these 33 repetitions are distributed, in a manner we cannot immediately determine from the profile, across the rest of the entries in the stages analysis. For the rest, we had 165 social utterances (see above) within the minor sentence-type, plus 51 instances of single-element sentences, as illustrated in the following extract:

T	'what are they dòing/
P	'talking
T	m̀hm/
P	'man

T   m̊hm/
P   ¯little gírl/ yès/[2]

Here, the first and second reponses of Mr J were single-element sentences. Notice (under the heading 'Statement') that 'nouns' (42) were much more common than 'verbs' (8) in this type of sentence; this is an important point, to which we shall return below.

In addition, there were 27 other sentences (both full and elliptical) which consisted of 2 or more elements and which could therefore be stated in terms of clause and/or phrase structure. It turned out that all of these fell into the category of statements. (The only possible instance of a nonstatement in the data was in the novel utterance quoted above *little gírl*. On the whole it seemed wisest to regard this conservatively, as a statement which has uncertain, slightly rising intonation.)

When we came to analyse those sentences which showed clause- and/or phrase-level structure, we found that there were in all 11 two-element constructions: one was an instance of SV, with a single phrase-level element realizing each of the clause-level elements S and V; two were VO (with the V consisting in each case of Aux + v); and 7 consisted of two phrase-level elements. In addition, there were 11 instances of three-element constructions which had the following form:

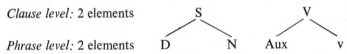

Clause level: 2 elements   S   V

Phrase level: 2 elements   D   N   Aux   v

In each case the clause-level element was expanded at phrase level as DN; and the phrase-level expansion of clause-level V was Aux and v. There were also two instances of three-element constructions at clause level (SVO), and one of a three-element construction at phrase level (DAdjN). Three occurrences of *and* at phrase-level (symbolized as c) were found in the sample: once followed by a single-phrase element, twice conjoining 2 Ns. The final point to notice at phrase level was the 14 instances of the use of some auxiliary verb—a feature which is characteristic of the three-element stage of normal first-language development. Together with this we took the 24 instances of *-ing* verb forms (in the word-level column), and noted the presence of a number of other word suffixes.[3]

This really concludes our examination of the first syntactic profile, which we have gone into in some detail. It was necessary to do this in order to prepare the ground for a description of the therapy programme which we subsequently followed. Now, however, it is profitable to take a few steps back, and put the profile—particularly the stages analysis—into perspective. We notice at once the unbalanced distribution of our observed constructions and single-element forms: the majority of major sentence types are found under 'N' at Stage I (42/79); and when we look for sentences with more than one element, we find relatively few entries at clause level, more at phrase level, and still more at word level. This

---

[2] ˭ indicates a held sound or syllable, often implying some articulatory difficulty.

[3] Interestingly, we found at this point just those which seem to occur earliest in normal first language development: the later, contracted forms, *'s*, *'cop*, *'aux*, and the comparative construction involving *-er*, had to be systematically introduced in the subsequent therapy schedule.

general pattern cuts across the postulated normal first-language developmental sequence, but we should not be surprised at this—rather the reverse; however, it clearly highlights the areas that needed immediate attention at the start of the therapy schedule, and we found that developmental norms proved most fruitful as an indication of the way in which the therapy schedule was to be subsequently maintained and developed.

The following extracts may help to indicate the nature of Mr J's language control at this stage (from session 1):

T	'what's thìs/ —	*showing picture of*
P	erm —	*cowboy lassoing*
T	mhḿ/ —	*horse*
P	'cowboys *'and —	
T	*mhḿ/ — —	
P	'cowboy 'and	*soft,*
	wréstler/ —	*slow*
	'wrestler 'and —	
T	wèll/ . the 'horse is 'tied with a rópe/ . ĭsn't it/	
P	a ròpe/ . 'ah 'yes yès/	
T	'what are they 'doing with the ròpe/ —	
	'what are they 'doing with the ròpe/	*soft*
P	strīng/ .	
T	ḿhm/ .	
P	yēs/ — —	
	strīng/ . strìng/	
T	mhḿ/ .	
	'they're pùlling it/	
P	pūl'ling 'it/ . 'ah yēs/ 'pu [*whispers*]	
T	*pùlling it/ .	
	*pùlling it/	
P	yès yes/	
	. . .	
T	'what are they dòing/ — —	
P	bōy/	
T	*mhḿ/ .	
P	*gīrl/ .	
T	mhḿ/ —	
	'try 'joining it ùp/ —	
P	*4 sylls.*	
T	'ah hăh/	
P	'the 'boy īs/	
T	goòd/ . ḿhm	
P	'the 'boy īs — —	
	'the 'boy īs — —	
	yĕs/ —	
	yĕs/	
T	rìght/ yĕs/ . you've gòt it/	
	sìtting/	

P	s̄īng it/	*soft*
	yēs	
T	sìtting	
P	*1 syll.*	
T	trý it/	
	lísten/	
	sìtting/ . sìtting/	
P	s̄īng . —	
T	the 'boy 'is *sìtting/	
P	*s̄īng —	
T	it 'won't come oùt/ will it/	
P	'‭t‬he 'boy 'is s̄ìtt.*ing/	
T	*ting/	
	gòod/	

The therapy procedure: aims and techniques

There was little room for argument as to what to do next, once the syntactic profile had been examined; clearly, clause-level structures had to be built up, at least to Stage III, with equivalent phrase-level consolidation, before anything else could be attempted. Then, we would be in a position to do something about the gaps in the Command and Question columns; we felt that commands and questions had priority over exclamations since they would help Mr J to use language in normal social situations, inside and outside the home, as soon as possible. At that point, we would review the situation, and work out a further stage in the remediation procedure.

However, we felt that it was worth while spending two more exploratory sessions with Mr J before starting the therapy schedule in earnest. There were two main questions to be approached: the first was that, as noted above (p. 166), rather few of the single-element sentences consisted of 'verbs', and we saw our task of developing clause-level structures as crucially dependent on the V category (see chapter 6); accordingly, we wanted to see how far V elements could be elicited at all. The second reason was that we wanted to investigate the possibility that Mr J's relative lack of multi-element constructions might be the result of an inability to control multi-syllabic sequences beyond a certain critical length. There was also the additional advantage of being able to assess, fairly informally, how stable Mr J's language ability was at this stage, and hence how representative the first syntactic profile was. As it turned out, these next two sessions provided us with fairly clearcut answers to our queries. As far as syllabic sequencing is concerned, we found that Mr J's relatively minor articulatory difficulties could not be held accountable for his lack of syntactic complexity—he was able to handle section C.4 of the Minnesota Test with very little difficulty, falling down only on the items *light the lamp* ([laɪt lə lamp]) and *easy does it* ([iːzi dʌd ɪz]). So we felt reasonably confident that his trouble was principally located at the level of syntax, as the profile suggested. Interestingly, the answer to our first question—how far could we elicit verbs, even in single-element utterances—put the relationship of Mr J's articulatory and syntactic difficulties in a new perspective for us; for, while it proved encouragingly possible to elicit verbs, we noted that V-function (as opposed to S/O/C function) at the level of syntax tended to increase the likelihood of articulatory problems, even over exactly the same phonological sequence. Thus, for example, the word *comb* as S/O/C presented no articulatory difficulty, but when Mr J was pressed to use it as a V, he at once started to lose articulatory control:

T	'what is she dòing/ —	
P	yès yes/ —	
	erm —	
	'the 'girl 'is . 'c̄omb . 'c̄o .	
	'the 'boy 'is .	*soft*
T	cómbing/	
P	còmbing/	
	yès yes/	
T	còmbing/	

We now began to consider the possibility that even the articulatory problems might, to some degree at least, be cleared up by intensive work on syntax (i.e. just the reverse of thinking that the syntax should wait upon phonological work). Of course, we recognized even at this stage that syntax was only one factor precipitating the articulatory problem; word-finding difficulties also aggravated it and we shall have more to say on this subject below. It looked, therefore, as if Mr J's articulation was generally good as long as his confidence (in handling language material especially) was undisturbed; we subsequently noted many occasions on which articulatory problems seemed to arise as a secondary result of trying to control something too difficult at the level of syntax; or of word-finding difficulties and consequent disturbed sentence structure; or of general low spirits.

It is worth pointing out here perhaps that Mr J generally had very good control of intonation (see what was said earlier regarding the use of *yes* and *no*) and relied on this a great deal at this time in order to communicate with his family and with T.

		demonstrates
T	'what's this when Ī'm —	*eating action*
	Ī'm/	
P	erm —	
	òh/ —	
T	'I ām/ —	
	'd'you 'get my . erm . àctions/	
	I've 'got a 'piece of 'cake and I'm —/	
	'maybe my àctions 'aren't very 'good/	
	try *thìs one/	
P	*nò no no/	
	mê/	
T	nò/ well* I .	
P	*nò no no/	
	mê/	
	nò no no/	

We discovered very quickly that whenever loss of intonational control occurred it provided a reliable indication of temporary loss of comprehension, or of inability to grasp the structure of a syntactic combination appropriately.

Subsequent to these two sessions (nos. 2 and 3), T fell ill for three weeks, and so the start of the therapy procedure was further delayed. However, it was encouraging to note that Mr J apparently retained a lot of the verbs material used in these sessions during this period; lack of retention had always been a major problem with him, according to the earlier therapists he had been assigned to.

The therapy procedure took as its first concern the task of building up basic SV and SVO patterns. For this purpose T used pictures (e.g. of a man digging, or a girl sewing a dress), in association with specific forms of questions (which we shall say something about in a moment). The idea was to progress from single-element elicited forms (we are talking all the time here of clause-level elements, each of which may have more than one phrase-level element realizing it), where the single element might be S, O or V; then on to two-element constructions of the form SV or VO; and eventually to three-element constructions of SVO form. We considered it important to use verbs such as *sewing, digging, eating, smoking* etc. since they have the very convenient property of functioning either with or without a direct object (O) (see chapter 6). The virtue of this is that it was possible for T to hold V constant for both SV and VO forms of the two-element sentence type; and to continue with the same V when proceeding to the three-element type. In this way we hoped to maximize the benefit gained from working on SV and VO separately when it came to fusing them. It may be useful to set out this discussion as follows:

	Elicited forms (clause-level elements)		
Step 1	Single element	S/O	= ((D)N) (*a*) *man* (*a*) *dress* etc.
		V	*digging, sewing* etc.
Step 2	Two elements	SV	*the man is digging* *the girl is sewing* etc.
		VO	*digging the garden,* *sewing a dress* etc.
Step 3	Three elements	SVO	*the man is digging the garden,* *the girl is sewing a dress* etc.

Now, in order to elicit these elements, both singly and in combinations, T had recourse to three principle types of stimulus (see chapter 6): the 'open discussion' type is illustrated by the following examples:[4]

---

[4] The desired responses are indicated in each case after the arrow; = shows the phrase-level structure of clause-level elements; > indicates progressively more complex responses as remediation continued. Types (*a*) to (*c*) are relatively simple, while (*d*) was reserved for a later stage in remediation.

> *1(a)* 'who is in this picture/   (→S (=(D)N))
>   *(b)* 'what is he/she dòing/   (→V (> VO > SVO))
>   *(c)* 'what is she sèwing/   (→O (=(D)(N))
>   *(d)* 'tell me about this pìcture/   (→SV/SVO)

The second consists of providing a list of alternatives, with no intonational cueing as to how large the set of alternatives may be (we refer to these as 'open alternatives'):

> *2(a)* is it a mán/ or a gírl/ or . . . etc.
>   *(b)* is she éating/ or drínking/ or . . . etc.

Finally, there is the 'forced alternatives' technique, occasionally extended to include more than two alternatives:

> *3(a)* is it a mán/ or a bòy/
>   *(b)* is he drínking/ or éating/ or smòking/
>   *(c)* is he 'eating an ápple/ or 'smoking a pìpe/

Both open alternatives (OA) and forced alternatives (FA) supplemented the open-discussion type of stimulus and were called on by T only when required; moreover, FA was used only when OA failed to elicit a response. In general, it was found that FA had to be used consistently at the start of the programme; one measure of progress was the ability of T gradually to fall back more and more on OA, and then to open discussion, and still elicit fully structured responses (although *1(a)*, *(c)* of course, as expected, tended to yield single clause-element responses). The eventual efficacy of *1(d)* to this end was taken to be an encouraging sign of successful therapy, since it represented the most open type of stimulus possible (that is, involving least structuring on the part of T). As a further point on elicitation techniques, and on FA in particular, it should be noted that a three-term FA (FA_3)—see *3(b)*— makes greater demands on P than a two-term (FA_2). This is for two main reasons: first, there is the simple consideration that the chance of guessing the right alternative drops straight away; but, secondly, we have also noted in some Ps, especially those with apparent short-term memory impairment, a definite tendency to select the last presented term (a recency effect), or the first presented term (an initial effect). In such cases, T, by using FA_3, may 'bury' the appropriate term in the middle whenever this procedure seems appropriate.[5] The distinction between *3(b)* and *3(c)*, with the latter including both V and O within the FA domain is an important point, but one that will be more conveniently taken up shortly.

Summary of therapy procedure

Before going on to give a detailed account of the main points of the therapy procedure, it is desirable to give a broad outline of the work that it was possible to get done in the first eight months of therapy, from September to May. As will be seen, the picture is not an entirely straightforward one:

---

[5] In general, we found FA_3 sufficient for this purpose; no apparent advantage was found with a four-term FA technique over OA.

Date	Session	Work done	Comments
25 Sept.	1	Exploratory: attempts to stimulate spontaneous speech using pictures + questions.	First syntactic profile done.
2 Oct.	2	Syllable sequencing (including phrases from Schuell); verb elicitation via actions.	
9 Oct.	3	Recap on sequencing; then on verbs; some work on new verbs.	Therapist ill; 3-week gap.
2 Nov.	4	FA work on V, N, Adj; → V, → S, → O, then → SV, → VO, → SVO.	
9 Nov.	5	FA on V + O; FA on 3 verbs; mass/ count nouns; *she is* > *she's* etc.	
16 Nov.	6	Recap SVO; spontaneous SVAs; reinforcement attempts; commands (*open/close* etc.)	Spontaneous use of SVO at home. Impending operation.
23 Nov.	7	Continue commands; adverbial/prepositional function of *in/on*; more commands.	Operation postponed.
—	—	Seen in ward 3 times; recap. of introduction of requests (*May I have* . . .).	Operation performed; success; no regression.
7 Dec.	8	Recap requests; *up/down* + *come/go* in adverbial and prepositional function; clause connection.	
14 Dec.	9	Concentration on directional (vs. relational) contrasts; *to/from*.	
21 Dec.	10	Recap of prepositions/adverbs; introduction of questions (*Where* . . .)	Starting to slow down.
11 Jan.– 1 Feb.	11/12	Only two sessions attempted, both unrecorded.	Christmas break. Depression.
8 Feb.	13	Recap SV, VO, SVO; sequencing	No confidence.
15 Feb.	14	FA work on pictures; then open questions; finally Adj (*full/empty*).	Much improved. Mild fit on 17 Feb.; but no regression.
22 Feb.	15	More work on Adj; → neg; attempts at SV → neg (not successful).	Second syntactic profile done.
1 Mar.	16	Neg with Adj; *unhappy* → *not happy*	
8 Mar.	—	Consultant's report; great improvement physically and linguistically.	Growing confidence.
15 Mar.	17	Adj → neg; SV → neg; SVO → neg.	
5 Apr.	18	Revision, mainly SVO; conjoined structures with *and*; linear sequencing better.	Third syntactic profile done.

Date	Session	Work done	Comments
19 Apr.	19	Conjoined structures, *and* → *then*; sequencing; questions.	
26 Apr.	20	Picture sequences, with written material; elaboration of structures over the same material.	
3 May	21	Further elaboration; two dimensions of structuring of written material.	Joins Red Cross Club.
10 May	22	Adverbials, with picture sequences; SV → SVA.	
17 May	23	Adverbials continued; SVO → SVOA.	
24 May	24	As for 23; FA resorted to.	Difficulty with *how/what* stimuli; materials problem.
31 May	25	More -*ly* adverbs; FA on new material.	Good spontaneous production.

As already pointed out, the procedure itself was begun in earnest only on session 4 after a gap of three weeks; thereafter, work progressed quite smoothly down to Christmas. Mr J responded well to FA work on building up clause structures, and T moved on fairly quickly (starting in session 6) to work on commands, followed by requests and questions. The idea here was to give sufficient language ability to Mr J as soon as possible to allow him to resume an active role within his family. Fortunately, no serious problems were encountered, in spite of the worry and disturbance attendant upon an operation (postponed once) for a haemorrhoids condition. However, a fall-off in Mr J's ability to take in new material was noticed in the last session (number 10) before the Christmas break; and this led into a period of depression which still had not lifted by 11 January (when session 11 was attempted). Both sessions 11 and 12 were necessarily outside the scope of the therapy procedure; T was mainly concerned to explore what was wrong, and to try to determine whether continued therapy would be of any benefit. This period of uncertainty continued up to and beyond 8 February when session 13, involving a recapitulation of basic work done before Christmas, was attempted. By session 14, Mr J was showing signs of willingness to accept further work, and of a growing confidence in his speech once more. This remained so even through a mild fit on 17 February, so much so that it proved possible on the next session (number 15, 22 February) to work out a second syntactic profile (see p. 174), as a guideline for subsequent remediation. This involved work with adjectives, and attempts at the development of clausal negation. On 5 April the third syntactic profile (see p. 175) was made and the latest stage of the programme, leading up to the introduction of adverbial elements, was implemented; after that time, he continued to progress fairly steadily in spite of a further mild fit (in July). He started to get out of the house much more than formerly, on grocery errands etc. He was also introduced into a local Red Cross club, where he met a variety of

A | **Unanalysed** | **Problematic**

1 Unintelligible **9**	2 Symbolic Noise	3 Deviant
1 Incomplete **51**	2 Ambiguous	

B **Responses**

Stimulus Type		Totals	Repet-itions	Elliptical Major 1	2	3	4	Full Major	Minor	Struc-tural	Ø	Prob-lems
61	Questions	**37**	**4**	**6**	**7**			**10**	**14**		**2**	
122	Others	**84**	**17**	**15**	**3**			**31**	**35**			

Normal Response / Abnormal

C **Spontaneous** **6** | **6** Others

Stage I (0;9–1;6) — Sentence Type

Minor **49**		Social **49**	Stereotypes	Problems
Major **78**		Sentence Structure		
Excl.	Comm.	Quest.	Statement	
	'V' **14**	'Q' 'V' **13** 'N'	Other Problems	

			Conn.	Clause		Phrase		Word

Stage II (1;6–2;0)

	V X	Q X		SV **9**	V C/O **10**	DN **86**	VV	-ing **68**
				S C/O	A X	Adj N **1**	V part	pl
				Neg X	Other	NN	Int X	
						PrN	Other	-ed

Stage III (2;0–2;6)

	V X Y	Q X Y	X + S:NP **7**	X + V:VP **9**	X + C/O:NP **10**	X + A:AP		-en
	let X Y	VS	SVC/O **32**	VC/OA	D Adj N **3**	Cop **2**		3s **46**
	do X Y		SVA	VO$_d$O$_i$	Adj Adj N	Aux **44**		gen
			Neg X Y	Other	Pr DN	Pron **3**		
					N Adj N	Other		

Stage IV (2;6–3;0)

	+ S	QVS	XY + S:NP **31**	XY + V:VP **30**	XY + C/O:NP **28**	Y + A:AP		n't
		QXYZ	SVC/OA	AAXY	N Pr NP	Neg V		'cop
			SVO$_d$O$_i$	Other	Pr D Adj N	Neg X		'aux
					cX	2 Aux		
					XcX	Other		

Stage V (3;0–3;6)

	how	tag	and	Coord. 1	1 +	Postmod. 1 clause	1 +	-est
	what		c	Subord. 1	1 +			-er
			s	Clause: S		Postmod. 1 + phrase		
			Other	Clause: C/O				-ly
				Comparative				

(+)			(−)			
NP	VP	Clause	NP		VP	Clause

Stage VI (3;6–4;6)

Initiator	Complex	Passive	Pron	Adj seq	Modal	Concord
Coord		Complement	Det	N irreg	Tense	A position
					V irreg	W order
Other			Other			

Stage VII (4;6+)

Discourse		Syntactic Comprehension	
A Connectivity	it		
Comment Clause	there	Style	
Emphatic Order	Other		

Total No. Sentences **127**	Mean No. Sentences Per Turn **0.7**	Mean Sentence Length **2.6**

Mr J: Profile 2

A	Unanalysed				Problematic		
	1 Unintelligible **6**	2 Symbolic Noise		3 Deviant	1 Incomplete **59**	2 Ambiguous	**6**

B Responses

Stimulus Type		Totals	Repet-itions	Elliptical Major 1	2	3	4	Full Major	Minor	Struc-tural	Ø	Prob-lems
60	Questions	**36**	**8**	**13**	**5**			**6**	**12**		**5**	
162	Others	**106**	**19**	**24**				**38**	**44**		**4**	

(Normal Response / Abnormal spanning headers: Elliptical Major over columns 1–4; Full Major, Minor; Struc-tural, Ø under Abnormal)

C Spontaneous | **23** | **17** | **4** | Others **19**

	Minor **56**		Social **52**	Stereotypes **4**	Problems

Sentence Type

Major **109**			Sentence Structure		

Stage I (0;9–1;6)

Excl.	Comm.	Quest.	Statement		
	'V'	'Q'	'V' **16** ·N· **21**	Other **3**	Problems

			Conn.	Clause	Phrase	Word

Stage II (1;6–2;0)

	V X	Q X	SV **17**	VC/O **12**	DN **121**	VV	-ing **90** pl
			S C/O	A X	Adj N **2**	V part	
			Neg X	Other	NN	Int X	
					PrN	Other	

Stage III (2;0–2;6)

	V X Y		X + S:NP **13**	X + V:VP **13**	X + C/O:NP **11**	X + A:AP	-ed / -en
		Q X Y	SVC/O **35**	VC/OA	D Adj N **11**	Cop **3**	
	let X Y	VS	SVA **4**	VO$_d$O$_i$	Adj Adj N	Aux **79**	3s **82** gen
			Neg X Y	Other	Pr DN **4**	Pron	
	do X Y				N Adj N	Other	

Stage IV (2;6–3;0)

			XY + S:NP **37**	XY + V:VP **36**	XY + C/O:NP **30**	Y + A:AP **4**	n't
	+ S	QVS	SVC/OA	AAXY	N Pr NP	Neg V	'cop
		QXYZ	SVO$_d$O$_i$	Other	Pr D Adj N	Neg X	'aux
					cX	2 Aux	
					XcX	Other	

Stage V (3;0–3;6)

	how		and	Coord. **1**	**1 +**	Postmod. **1** clause	**1 +**	-est
		tag	c	Subord. **1**	**1 +**			-er
			s	Clause: S		Postmod. **1 +** phrase		
	what		Other	Clause: C/O				-ly
				Comparative				

(+)			(−)			
NP	VP	Clause	NP		VP	Clause

Stage VI (3;6–4;6)

Initiator	Complex	Passive	Pron	Adj seq	Modal	Concord
Coord		Complement	Det	N irreg	Tense	A position
					V irreg	W order
Other			Other			

Discourse		Syntactic Comprehension	

Stage VII (4;6 +)

A Connectivity	it		
Comment Clause	there	Style	
Emphatic Order	Other		

Total No. Sentences **165**	Mean No. Sentences Per Turn **0·7**	Mean Sentence Length **2·5**

© D. Crystal, P. Fletcher, M. Garman, 1975 University of Reading

Mr J: Profile 3

other patients (not all of them, of course, dysphasic). In August, when this chapter was written, he was again worried and depressed, this time at the prospect of being assigned to a new therapist. It was hoped and expected that this setback would prove to be temporary.

Details

In this section we want to highlight a number of points that came up during the schedule of remediation. The selection of these points has been guided by two considerations: first, we believe that, in spite of the diversity of language disabilities found in adult dysphasics generally, these points are liable to be encountered quite commonly when working in the area covered by a remediation schedule of the type being described here; secondly, they will conveniently serve as representative illustrations of the techniques and aims which have been discussed in rather more general terms above.

(*i*) Linear segmentation

A rather serious problem of linear segmentation, or the structuring of syntactic sequences, arose very early in remediation. Already by session 4, we observed the occurrence of SVO and SV structures where an abnormal intonational and rhythmic contour regularly appeared, and seemed to point to an inappropriate structuring on Mr J's part of the internal components of the sequence in question. For the SVO pattern, what would happen is illustrated by:

'the 'boy 'is . 'eating 'a . 'apple

 S   V   O

For SV structures, this has an even more disruptive effect:

T   whò is it/
P   'the 'man 'is . 'fishing 'a
T   wèll/ thàt's it/
        the 'man is fìshing/

Even S may be broken up in this way:

'the . 'girl . 'is . 'sewing a . 'dress

Notice in these cases how the pauses (.) fail to coincide with the boundaries of clause-level elements, suggesting that for Mr J the sequence consisted of three components which are not quite the same as S, V and O. In the first example, for instance, the first group includes *is* (which is typically accompanied by an abnormal degree of stress), while the second consists of the main verb followed by the indefinite article (part of O), which is also stressed. In this last case, one problem became apparent at once; the indefinite article was represented by its most widely distributed form *a*, whereas in fact *apple* requires the less frequent form *an*. If both the D and N elements of O had been encoded together, one would not have expected this problem to arise. However, if the indefinite article is encoded prior to selection of the N (of O), then this is exactly what one would predict. Equally, Mr J had problems regarding the auxiliary element (*is*) of V; the true relationship between S and V is such that the distribution of the singular/plural auxiliaries *is/are* in:

> The boy is eating
> The boys are eating

exactly parallels the distribution of the simple present forms of verbs (e.g. *eats/eat*), as in:

> The boy eats
> The boys eat.

But insofar as Mr J treated *is* (and presumably also *are*, where this occurred at all) as one with elements such as *the boy*, and as distinct from verbal elements, then it was likely that this important parallelism of singular and plural forms of V was going to be missed.

We said earlier (p. 169) that we would return to the matter of how far syntactic and lexical factors played a role in the articulatory ability of Mr J, and we noted the possibility that the syntactic difference between noun and verb function of a particular word (e.g. *comb*) might cause segmental phonological problems. Now, at this point we may see a possible effect of word-finding problems on the non-segmental phonological pattern. For what seemed to be happening was that pauses were breaking up the SVO pattern just at those points where major lexical choices had to be made. We hypothesized at the time along the following lines. Words such as *boy, eat, apple* are often treated, both traditionally and in more recent grammatical theory, as fundamentally different from words such as *a, the, is* etc.: the distinction has been given labels such as 'major'/'minor' words, 'open'/'closed' sets of words, 'full'/'open' words, 'lexical'/'grammatical' words. However difficult we may find it to define the boundary between these two types in a precise, once-for-all manner (cf. Crystal 1966), we immediately perceive the nature and practicality of such a distinction. One way to model the distinction is to visualize the grammar as containing a vocabulary component (or lexicon) in which full lexical items are stored and from which they can be selected and inserted into structures which are specified in the syntactic component. The syntactic component as well as containing rules for enumerating structures (SV, SVO, DN etc.), will also contain sets of grammatical words, which will already be specified in the syntactic structures, prior to the insertion of items from the lexicon. It must be stressed at this point that terms such as 'already' and 'prior to' in this very informal account, must not be taken at face value to imply temporal order; it is rather an article of faith with linguists that one can only impose a 'logical precedence' interpretation on the use of such terms, if they are to be used at all. This said, however, we feel that little harm is done in using them in this case; for it is observed that Mr J produced *is* considerably before (temporally) he produced the complex form *eating* (containing the major lexical item *eat*), and *a* likewise before the major item *apple*. It was precisely these temporal pauses that interrupted the intonation contour; and we may ask here if it might not be the case that two fundamental activities, lexical search and syntactic construction, are in fact temporally as well as procedurally related, in such a way that problems with the first of these tended to disturb the implementation of the second. Although there are many interpretations possible within this general position, we took the view that word-finding problems were resulting in an abnormal intonation pattern; and that this in turn may have been affecting the development of basic clause structure (by disrupting feedback from Mr J's own productions).

When the segmentation problem arose, we were seriously concerned to find a solution as soon as possible. Three main possibilities presented themselves straight away:

(a)   We might restrict the vocabulary as far as possible, so that Mr J could learn, by rote if necessary to begin with, which Vs required Os and which did not;[6]
(b)   We could work much more on the transition from SV and VO to SVO (keeping V constant over the three structures in each case);
(c)   We could reserve three-element structures until later on in the remediation programme, and concentrate on eliminating hesitation points in the S and V elements before proceeding.

However, all these possibilities had the attendant disadvantage of leading to an overuse of basically the same language material; and, while this is of course an important methodological problem with all patients, we suspect that it is usually particularly acute with adults, and certainly necessitated serious consideration as far as Mr J was concerned (see also p. 189). We therefore attempted indirect ways around the problem, of which, again, there were three:

(i)   We included V + O in the FA technique (see 3(c) above) as in:

is she 'sewing a dréss/ or 'eating a càke/

(ii)   We introduced contracted forms, via use of pronouns:

the . 'girl is . VÈRBing/
she is . VÈRBing/
she's VÈRBing/

(iii)   We alternated a(n)/the in the D position of O elements, and alternated also mass and count nouns in the N position of these elements:

$$\text{She's eating} \left\{ \begin{array}{l} \left\{ \begin{array}{l} \text{an} \\ \text{the} \end{array} \right\} \quad \begin{array}{l} \text{àpple} \\ \\ \text{soùp} \end{array} \end{array} \right\}$$

With (i), we hoped to develop in Mr J an awareness that V and O hang together in an SVO structure as a particularly cohesive unit; by supplying both major

---

[6] Cf. ch. 6 for reasons for the focus on VO.

lexical choices together (V and O) in each of the forced alternatives, we were able to elicit intonationally sound responses, which could serve as appropriate feedback. Clearly, this was just to get Mr J moving, as it were, and would not be appropriate over a long period. With (*ii*) we hoped first of all to eliminate the possibility of hesitation within the S; and then, by eliminating the Subject–Aux hesitation point, to make the Aux–Verb hesitation point the first one in the sentence; this might then be eliminated by encouraging Mr J to complete the first lexical choice prior to starting the utterance. Finally, with (*iii*) we wanted to highlight the dependency between D (*a(n)*/*the*), or lack of D, and the type of N that follows. We could, in principle, have extended this method by taking in plural count nouns (which, like non-count nouns, do not pattern with *a(n)*), but we felt that this might be counter-productive in possibly confusing Mr J. On the whole, methods (*i*) and (*ii*) proved to be the most successful; an example of (*ii*) is this:

T	whò's 'walking/
P	'the . 'girl is . w̄àlking/ yès/
T	gòod/
	sǒ/ shè's/ *wàlking/
P	*wàlking/ yès/
T	agaìn/
P	'she's wàlking/ *confidently*
T	'very goòd/

But wrong segmentation remained a serious problem right across the range of structures we wanted to produce, and was still not entirely cleared up at the time of writing; for example (from the session on command structures):

P	'put . 'back the . 'cigarettes pleăse/ —	*intake of breath*
	erm	
	'put . 'back the . ['attrĕɪ]/pleăse/ —	*ashtray*
	'put . 'back the . [àttrĕɪ] 'please/	*second ashtray*

(*ii*) Incipient structure

Up till now, we have talked as though the remediation procedure was implemented throughout as it had been conceived on the basis of the initial syntactic profile—albeit with modifications and supplementation in order to cope with such problems as the one regarding linear segmentation that has just been discussed. This may well be the usual case when one is working with young children, helping them to overcome a general or specific language delay; but when dealing with stroke patients (and probably adult dysphasics generally), one is always liable to encounter incipient structure (see pp. 116–17) at any level of description—phonological, syntactic, semantic. A case in point arose in session 6 when T was prepared to revise basic SV(O) structures prior to moving on to commands. What happened was a sudden emergence of adverbials during the revision of SVO, as is illustrated in the following transcription:

P   the 'girl is . 'sitting *dòwn/ yès/
T   *goòd/
       wèll done/
       goòd/

(*NB* T reinforces here just as P produces the unlooked-for adverbial *down.*)

. . .

P   the 'girl is . on her ówn/ yĕs/
T   goòd yes/ OK̂/

(P was uncertain of his control of the adverbial here, hence the rising intonation—as if to ask 'is this correct?')

. . .

P   the 'girl is . 'in . bèd/
T   rìght/

For T this was a particularly awkward—though naturally gratifying in a general way—point for incipient structure to arise, because it happened right at the start of the main commands > requests > questions component of the remediation procedure. We felt that such a progression would demand the full attention of both Mr J and T, and we were reluctant either to ignore or wholly follow the A-elements when they appeared in this unsolicited fashion.

In order to explain what we decided upon and why, we must first take a closer look at A-elements in English. At clause level, we may note that A-elements modify basic SV and SVO structures in the following principal ways:

		SV type		*SVO type*
(*a*)	SVA	John ate hungrily	SVOA	John ate the food hungrily
(*b*)	ASV	Hungrily, John ate	ASVO	Hungrily, John ate the food
(*c*)	SAV	John hungrily ate	SAVO	John hungrily ate the food

Of the three A positions here, (*a*) is traditionally recognized as basic: while (*b*) preserves the basic SV(O) pattern undisturbed, it carries an exceptional intonational contour (cf. the comma in orthographic representation), whereby the front A-element is emphasized; and (*c*) involves insertion of the A-element within the basic SV(O) structure (though we should notice in this example the impossibility of breaking up V and O in this way). At phrase level, *A grammar of contemporary English* makes the following classification of A-elements, which we list here for convenience:

(*i*)   Adverbials (most commonly, those ending in *-ly* as *hungrily, slowly, quickly* etc.)
(*ii*)   Noun phrases (e.g. *last week*)
(*iii*)   Prepositional phrases (e.g. *in September, in the garden, by stealth*)
(*iv*)   Finite clauses (e.g. *when he had finished*)

    (*v*) Nonfinite clauses

        (*a*) *-ing* (e.g. *waiting at the bus-stop*)

        (*b*) *to* (e.g. *to get the groceries*)

        (*c*) *-ed* (e.g. *terrified but determined*)

    (*vi*) Verbless clauses (e.g. *apologetic about everything*)

From this it may be appreciated that types (*iv*) to (*vi*) are more difficult than (*i*) to (*iii*), presupposing as they do a complex sentence structure. This is true even of type (*vi*) where the verb of the A-element clause has been elided. Moreover, of (*i*) to (*iii*), type (*ii*) constitutes a relatively small set; and we thought it best to concentrate first on introducing those structures which would have the greatest chance of common use. A further point of difficulty with using type (*ii*) was that we wanted to emphasize the distinctness of clause-level elements such as V, A, and S/O as much as possible, as an aid to Mr J's developing ability to structure them together; and using exponents of A which at phrase-level were not distinct from exponents of S/O was felt to be a possible source of confusion. This left us with types (*i*) and (*iii*), if we were to introduce A-elements at all. In this connection, it was encouraging that these were just the types that Mr J had spontaneously produced. In this light, we rethought the implications of our original therapy procedure (see p. 168), and noticed a point that probably should have occurred to us before: prior to developing commands, questions, and other socially important structures (e.g. requests), it is probably not enough simply to have reached the stage where P can handle basic SV(O) patterns (as in statements). For commands, questions etc. are not simply transformationally related versions of statements, but are inextricably bound up in their own particular situations, within which they are appropriate forms of linguistic behaviour, and require their own forms of linguistic or nonlinguistic response. Moreover, ability to handle any one of these types involves both production and comprehension; and very often these different types will be found to complement each other within a single dialogue. We can perhaps make these points clearer with some hypothetical but realistic examples:

    (*a*) Give me a cigarette. (*command*)

Responses $\begin{cases} \text{Tell me where you put them.} \quad (command) \\ \text{Are they in the kitchen?} \quad (question) \end{cases}$

    (*b*) Where are my cigarettes? (*question*)

Responses $\begin{cases} \text{Think where you last put them.} \quad (command) \\ \text{Did you leave them in the kitchen?} \quad (question) \end{cases}$

It is common experience that a simple command or question is not always going to achieve the desired effect, even with the most sympathetic listener; one particularly important supplementary piece of the dialogue is the command type (e.g. *Tell me where you put them*), and another is the question (e.g. *Did you leave them in the kitchen?*). Notice that with the first of these, the speaker ought to be able to supply the required information immediately, all as part of the overall command, or question—and for this he must be able to control A-elements (providing the precise location of the cigarettes, in this example) in his production. Equally, with questions from the addressee, the first speaker must be able to control A-elements (*in the kitchen?*) in his comprehension.

We therefore decided that what had emerged as incipient structure in Mr J's case was in fact relevant to the aims of our original procedure at this point; and we were also clear about the phrase-structure types that we wanted to introduce first. There was however one final consideration, which concerned our choice of particular lexical items in remediation, and this will be brought out in the next section.

(*iii*)   Adverbial/prepositional function

Thus far, we have discussed A-element types (*i*) adverbials and (*iii*) prepositional phrases as though there were no point of contact between them; but this is not really the case. At word-structure level (at which Mr J showed most control, once he had found the required lexical item) types (*i*) and (*iii*) are closely linked, through the class of items such as *up, down, in, over*, etc. These may function either as type (*i*) elements, as in:

```
The man   ran    up
The ball   went   down
    S        V      A
```

or as prepositions within type (*iii*) constructions, as in:

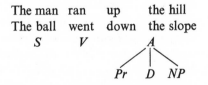

```
The man   ran    up      the hill
The ball   went   down    the slope
    S        V              A
                         ╱  │  ╲
                        Pr  D  NP
```

Now, given the possibility that we could introduce both type (*i*) and type (*iii*) patterns via the same lexical items (thus restricting the scope of the word-finding task), we were faced with the decision as to which pattern should be concentrated on first. We saw two advantages to treating type (*i*) as basic: first, the overall structure is shorter (i.e. by a whole NP): secondly, the degree of contrast between *up, down, in, over* etc. in adverbial function (type (*i*)) is often greater than that between the same elements in prepositional function (type (*iii*), and we thought that this would help Mr J in developing his A-elements system to begin with. The greater degree of contrast is partly the function of position within the whole structure; final position, which often seems to be reserved for information-bearing elements, is occupied by *up* in *The man ran up* (i.e. he didn't run *down*, or *across* or *over*); but it is occupied by *the hill* in *The man ran up the hill* (i.e. he didn't run up *the ladder*, or *the road*, or *the mountain*). However, we also saw the advantages of linking the two patterns as explicitly as possible, and aimed for a considerable period of overlap in their use in the remediation procedure; and the introduction of both patterns was made within the framework of the original schedule (involving commands, requests and questions).

T started off with commands involving a penny, and a box with reference to which the penny could be placed by Mr J in various locations. Thus Mr J had to comprehend not only the command structure, but also, in order to respond appropriately, the adverbial contrast (which was restricted initially to *in* versus *on*). T aimed, later on, to introduce questions in relation to commands (by asking *Where is the penny?* after a command had been appropriately responded to by Mr J), thereby also starting to switch roles of production and comprehension between Mr J and T; and, eventually, to get Mr J making the commands (and supplementary questions).

To begin with, there was little difficulty, and Mr J responded in the main with appropriate responses (nonverbal—simply placing the penny in/on the box). Then T started to ask Mr J for a verbal response to accompany the nonverbal (keeping it as simple as possible to begin with—*in* or *on*):

T	'listen to 'me first of ăll/ —
	òn the bóx/ —
	*ìn the 'box/
P	*ìn the 'box/ —
	òn the bóx/ —
	in the box/ yès/
T	'good for yôu/
	'well dône/
P	yès yes/

But trouble came when Mr J, having correctly placed the penny (on the box, in this instance) and correctly described his action, was subsequently unable to describe its location (*NB* using the prepositional function); this was the case even though T reverted to FA at this point:

T	nòw/ 'put it òn the 'box/
P	òn the 'box/ yès/
T	rìght/
	*goòd/
P	*yès/
T	nòw/ 'where ìs it/ —
	is it ìn the box/ or òn the 'box/ nòw/
P	in the bóx/ . nò/ . òn the bóx/ . nŏ/

A short while after (in the same session) T again approached this area, working towards a complete SVA. At first, there was some success:

T	can we 'have the 'whole thìng/
P	òn the 'box/
T	mhm̀/
	thĕ/ —
P	the . 'penny is òn the 'box/

T   wéll dòne/
        agaìn/
P   the 'penny is 'on the bòx
T   agaĭn/
P   'the . 'penny is 'on the bòx/ .

but it was lost again shortly afterwards:

P   the . 'penny ĭs/ — —
        the . 'penny ĭs/. — —
        the . — — —
        shut the doòr/ (*laughs*)

(*Shut the door* is a wellworn routine from earlier sessions on command structures, put in here for humorous effect by Mr J, acknowledging his inability to supply what is required.)

Whatever was wrong at this point seemed to be specific to elements such as *in/on*, since the session (no. 7) as a whole was successful in other ways (see the discussion of commands, below), and Mr J was working cheerfully and well. Apparently we had reached the point of satiation as far as *in/on* were concerned; and we therefore reconsidered our choice of lexical items for adverbial work. As a result, we concluded that *in/on* were too close to each other, semantically (and perhaps phonologically too): they both referred to location of X at Y (with the *in/on* distinction referring to different modalities of 'being at'); and, in the way that we had been using them, they both referred to stable schemata, encoded as 'stative' linguistic patterns.[7] In particular, it is probably important to note that *on* can be used in very general 'contact' situations, as in even *The fly is on the ceiling* (not *under/beneath the ceiling*).

Accordingly, in the next session, T used *up/down* in dynamic constructions. It should be noted here that *up/down* are in contrast along two possible dimensions, which we may call the 'relational' (stative) and the 'directional' (dynamic). Thus, on the first of these, we have:

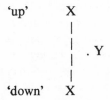

—which simply means that *X is up/down* makes sense only in relation to some reference point Y (which may be an earlier position of X). On the second dimension, it is the direction of travel (dynamic) that forms part of the relevant opposition as is shown by the arrows:

[7] On the distinction between 'stative' and 'dynamic', and for the relationship between *in* and *on*, see Lyons 1968, 324–5.

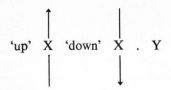

'up' X 'down' X . Y

Here also, of course, some reference point is required, to distinguish movement up from movement down.

Essentially the same point has to be made about *in/out*, which T dealt with after *up/down*; we shall briefly consider the two dimensions of this opposition here, before going on to show its relevance for the way therapy was conducted for Mr J. In the case of *in/out*, the stative opposition may be pictured as:

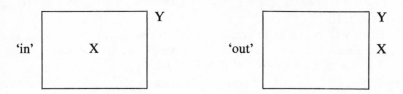

Notice that we again need the reference point Y, which in this instance has to be able to contain X. Now, the dynamic opposition may be pictured in two ways:

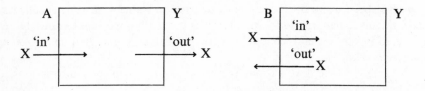

Notice that in both A and B *in* refers to movement from a position like that for stative *out*, to a position like that for stative *in*, and vice versa. Now, in A the direction of travel from one position to another is constant with reference to Y; but in B it is reversed between *in* and *out*. So, in A we can say that there is movement which results in an opposition of location which is essentially like the stative opposition; while in B there is an opposition of *movement* (directional) which leads to a stative opposition of location. Or again, there are *two* oppositions in B, but only *one* in A.

Now, in order to emphasize the dynamic contrast, we originally decided to link *up/down* (which T worked on first) to directionally-opposed verbs of the most basic type in English, viz. *come/go*. Thus, T always used *go + up*, and *come + down* (in the context of rockets going to the moon and returning to earth etc.). Our first discovery was not long in coming: Mr J at once, and quite reasonably, ignored this arbitrary pairing, and seemed quite unhelped by our attempt to keep the directional opposition constant in both V and A. He handled structures like the following very well:

This $\begin{Bmatrix} \text{rocket} \\ \text{bus} \end{Bmatrix}$ is $\begin{Bmatrix} \text{going} \\ \text{coming} \end{Bmatrix}$ up

This $\begin{Bmatrix} \text{rocket} \\ \text{bus} \end{Bmatrix}$ is $\begin{Bmatrix} \text{going} \\ \text{coming} \end{Bmatrix}$ down

Notice the use of *this* as D; Mr J seemed to have no trouble in taking this over from T's own description of the drawings that were used for this part of the procedure. Having got this far, T now explored the possibility of eliciting prepositional function of *up/down* (*NB* keeping the tone contrast on *up/down*):

This bus is $\begin{Bmatrix} \text{going ùp} \\ \text{coming dòwn} \end{Bmatrix}$ the hill.

This proved no problem, and we felt that we might well have succeeded, or be in process of succeeding, as far as our two main aims were concerned: first, to consolidate incipient structure of the A type, and secondly, to link these two A categories by introducing them systematically together. Moreover, it was noticeable at this point that Mr J's good intonational control was starting to modify the intonation of the opposing structures (linking them into a single intonational unit):

This bus is going úp (the hill); this bus is going dòwn (the hill).

The parentheses indicate that this was true of both adverbial and prepositional function of *up/down*; and we were so encouraged by this that we decided to treat it as ripe for consolidation too, and introduced the conjunction *and*. We hoped in this way to capitalize on our work with incipient structure at phrase level by using it as a natural framework within which to build up still more clause-level complexity. Interestingly, the distinction between adverbial and prepositional function came out most clearly here, and in the expected direction; Mr J could handle conjunction of two adverbial function patterns, but prepositional function proved too much:

P	'this 'rocket 'is 'going ǔp/ ǎnd/ . *'this 'rocket 'is 'going dòwn/
T	*rǐght/
...	
P	'this 'bus 'is . 'going . ùp the 'hill/
T	gǒod/
P	'this 'bus 'is . gōing/ . nòw/ — 'the . yès/ — —
T	mhm̀/
P	'this 'bus . 'is . 'going . dòwn/ . 'the . hǐll/.
T	rǐght/
P	ǎnd/ . 'this . 'bus . 'is . 'going . 'down the hîll/ 'yes — 'the — — —
T	'which 'one is going dòwn/ shòw me/ which one/

P   ùp/   *pointing*
T   that's rĭght/ ŭp/ ānd/
P   dòwn/
T   dòwn/ yès/ goòd/
P   ŭp/. ănd/. dòwn/
T   goòd/.

Notice how here the adverbial function of *up/down* still elicits an appropriate response. It may be that sentence length is the limiting factor here: but, as we pointed out earlier, it is confounded with vaguer notions such as degree of semantic contrast, which may be at least equally important.

Two final points may be made here. The first, which takes up the issue introduced above, concerning *in/out*, shows the importance of directional opposition; T had been using *in/out* in connection with a dog and a kennel where the movement of the dog was constant:

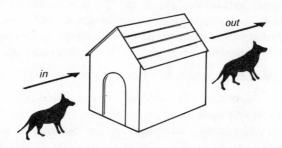

(Clearly, this kennel had a back door!) Mr J found this problematic, rather to our surprise: his production of *in/out* descriptions showed uncertain intonation, long pauses and occasional loss of the opposition (even for adverbial functions of *in/out*). At length, Mr J took the rubber stamp which T was using, for depicting the dog, and experimented for a while, eventually coming up with the following:

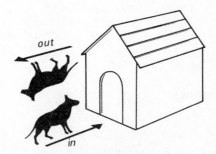

He was then able to say *in* and *out* confidently (pointing to the appropriate dog), and seemed much happier with this revised schema—even though one of the rubber-stamp dogs was now necessarily upside down.[8] He was subsequently able

---

[8] Assuming that the dog had always to be facing in the direction of its travel, rather than moving backwards—which seems reasonable enough.

to produce full structures involving both adverbial and prepositional function of *in/out* (*NB out of* is the complex prepositional group which corresponds to the adverbial *out*). We are convinced that Mr J was in effect highlighting here the importance of the directional contrast (rather than, say, objecting to the notion that kennels have back doors), since exactly the same modification was required later on in the session in respect of two trains and a tunnel (one going in, the other coming out).

The second, and last, point is that this excursus into A-elements at phrase and word level at once started to yield a limited productivity, and this has steadily improved ever since. The first instance that we noted was the following:

P	the 'boy is . [ɒpskɑʃ]/ yés/	'hopscotch'
T	wĕll/	
P	yès yes yes/	*humorously*
T	yès/	*laughing*
P	the 'boy is . 'hopscotch . plàying/	
	the 'boy is . 'playing . 'with a . hòpscotch/	
	yès yes/	*laughing*
T	'jolly gòod/ OǨ/ rìght/	

Given the close relation between:

$$\text{X plays with a} \begin{Bmatrix} \text{football} \\ \text{volleyball} \end{Bmatrix}$$

and

$$\text{X plays} \begin{Bmatrix} \text{football} \\ \text{volleyball} \end{Bmatrix}$$

we were not too worried by this. The main concern was to get Mr J's syntax moving again, and to leave finer matters regarding the boundary of syntax and semantics to a much later date. We were confident, for example, that an utterance such as:

the 'boy is . foòtball/

did not indicate that Mr J thought that a particular boy was a football. Perhaps the most encouraging point regarding the hopscotch example was the degree of self-correction that was involved.

(iv) The plateau

It is convenient at this point to say something about the difficulty that Mr J showed in taking in structured therapy, from 21 December to 15 February. T had had considerable success in introducing command structures, leading to requests, and was now approaching questions; and, as has been discussed above, definite progress was being made simultaneously with A-elements. We decided that, in view of the problems in conjoining structures such as:

This bus is going úp the hill
This bus is going dòwn the hill,

it would be as well to avoid further clause-level complexity of this type; it might well prove more suitable to build up *and-* constructions from phrase-level first (*red and green pen* > *red pen and green book*; *running up and down* > *running up and walking down*). T therefore decided to focus on *wh-* questions in the session on 21 December (number 10); this being the last session before the Christmas break, we looked forward to being able to complete the introduction of all the major structures in this first part of the remediation procedure. It should also be said, however, that we were conscious of the need to move on as soon as possible to new material and fresh structures: Mr J was understandably showing distinct signs of boredom with the material involved with *in/out, up/down* etc. We naturally wanted to concentrate our efforts mainly on those structures which would socialize him as rapidly as possible.

This session was the first one where T was accompanied by one of the authors; Mr J's relatively poor performance in this session was at first put down to this potentially disturbing influence, but we later revised our opinion about this, as will be seen below. After a brief warm-up on familiar material (involving *up/down*)— where Mr J's ability was noticeably down on the previous session—T started introducing *wh-* questions, concentrating mainly on the *wh-* word *where*. The first part of this introduction involved a comprehension task only—and this seemed to be perfectly good as far as his vision extended: he was able to point and say *There, On the table* etc. to questions such as *Where is the TV?* The next stage required Mr J to ask T where various objects in the room were. Here the same sort of problem was encountered as when in session 7 he had had to command his daughter to perform certain actions (*Bring the ash-tray*, for example): he often responded with the answer instead of asking the question. (With commands, he had initially tended to perform the action instead of commanding it.) In an effort to overcome this, T and Mr J joined together as a question-asking team, with Mr J's wife and daughter, and the author who was present, as a question-responding team. T was now able to provide model question structures where necessary without Mr J's assuming that they were genuine questions rather than models. However, there remained a great deal of uncertainty on Mr J's part; wrong linear segmentation was particularly noticeable in his production, as was a shaky grasp of intonational structure. Moreover, we also found that he could often only initiate a question structure with the name of the object whose location was being questioned; and he would repeat this word until T showed him the word *where* (written in block letters on a card), whereupon the whole structure would be produced:

T	'what tèlevision/ 'you ask Mĭke/	
P	Mĭke/ . télevision/	
T	nŏw/ re'member 'how we are àsking it/	
P	yès/	
	Mĭke/	*T shows card*
	'where is the . télevision/	
T	'where is the tèlevision/	
P	'where is the tèlevísion/	

In general during this session, it appeared that word-finding difficulties were tending to displace Mr J's attention to syntactic structure; and there was very little carryover even from one part of the session to the other. Material that had eventually been successfully handled after initial difficulties apparently presented exactly similar difficulties when re-presented only a few minutes later on.

When T returned, after the Christmas break, Mr J was still generally depressed and unwilling to work through further therapy; at this stage it was an open question as to whether this was a period of regression or simply a 'plateau'. T maintained friendly social contact—and, on a couple of occasions, arrived without a tape-recorder and was surprised by Mr J who insisted that a therapy session be conducted! However, these were relatively ineffectual sessions from the point of view of the past performance of Mr J, and of the expectations embodied in the therapy programme.

(v) The development of negative structures

Eventually, however, T was able to make a serious revision of basic SV, VO and SVO structures (session 13, 8 February), and to proceed from there to an elicitation task involving description of well-known routines or action sequences such as lighting a cigarette, plugging in and operating a tape-recorder etc. Mr J showed great willingness to cooperate, and a fair amount of retention; but his control of intonation patterns was shaky, and he generally showed a marked lack of confidence. In an effort to introduce as much variety as possible into the therapy materials, T went on in the next session to work with picture-lotto material which it was hoped would prove to be both graphically simple and yet unchildish. T progressed from FA to open questions on this material, and Mr J showed much improved confidence and interest. Finally, T introduced adjectives, relying for the most part on contrast between pairs (such as *big/small, tall/short, full/empty* etc.) for ease of acquisition. Adjectives were felt to be a suitable area to work on at this stage for the following reasons: first, the first syntactic profile showed rather little SVC clause structure (*the ball is red*), and few instances of Adj-types at phrase level; secondly SVC clause structure was a natural extension of SVO structure and should therefore cause little difficulty even though it represented new material; thirdly, linking SVC structures (*the ball is red*) to corresponding phrase structures (*the red ball . . .*) would allow simultaneously for development of language control at two levels, and, we hoped, would allow Mr J to intuit the regular relationship between the two. In this connection, it should be noted that we followed general linguistic thought in taking SVC function of adjectives to be basic, and noun phrasal function (prenominal modification) to be derived from this. Finally, we felt that, having established adjectives (proceeding from clause structure to phrase structure), we could use this framework for the introduction of negative structures (proceeding from lexical negation and morphological negation and building up to clause level—cf. what was noted above on p. 186 regarding the operation of the conjunction *and*). This was, of course, an important component of our original programme of therapy for the post-Christmas period.

Accordingly, after T had asked questions such as:

'is the 'girl 'washing her fáce/

P provided fully structured responses quite regularly (though note the concord problem, which we did not attempt to grapple with at this stage):

P   yès/ the 'girl is 'washing his fàce/

T then moved on to general adjectives, as illustrated here:

T   is the 'dress pínk/ or grèen/ (*FA*) — —
       'what 'colour is the drèss/ (*open discussion*)
P   the 'dress is pìnk/

Subsequently she moved quickly on to contrasting adjective pairs, as in:

T   is the 'bottle fúll/ or èmpty/

Now, Mr J was picking up quite a lot of visual cues from the printed description of the pictures all through this session, so it was quite surprising to us that he showed unresolvable hesitation when faced with this question. In particular, we had reason to believe that up until now Mr J's word-finding difficulties had largely been circumvented by the use of such visual cues. Since *full/empty* may be characterized as positive/negative lexical items respectively, we were faced with the possibility that a quite separate problem from the word-finding one was being encountered here, having to do with negation. This suspicion was strengthened as a result of the following sort of situation, where T was simply testing comprehension of the negative term:

T   /is the 'bottle émpty/ (*of a full or empty bottle*)
P   /yés/ . nó/

By contrast, asking the positive version of the question generally prompted a single, definite response (as long as the bottle was full):

T   /is the 'bottle fúll/ (*of a full bottle*)
P   /yès/

If the depicted bottle was empty, Mr J would show the same hesitation as when he was asked the negative version of the question. It should be pointed out here that at this stage he was able to take (perfectly legitimate) evasive action when T tried to elicit a negative sentence structure; as an illustration of this, we may cite the following:

T   /is the 'cow stánding/ (*cow pictured lying down*)
P   /nǒ/ the 'cow is sìtting/

Notice here that, apart from the negative particle *no*, the sentence structure is positive, not negative; and that Mr J substituted a different lexical item (*sitting* for *standing* in T's structure). This is all the more remarkable in view of his word-finding problems, of course. Now, the difference between *standing/sitting* on the one hand and *full/empty* on the other is that only the latter pair is opposed as positive/negative. So we had the following situation at this stage: Mr J would resort to lexical substitution in order to avoid sentence negation, only so long as lexical negation was not involved. The problem was thus clearly one regarding negation itself, and seemed to arise equally with T's use of words such as *empty* and with the use of pictures showing an empty as opposed to a full bottle.

In the next session (number 15), T began with a revision of adjectives that had been fairly well handled the previous week, and then moved on to the problem of *full/empty* again. Whereas, however, the bottle depicted had previously been either full or empty, on this occasion T used a picture of a half-filled bottle (i.e. not characterized appropriately as either *full* or *empty*). We did not seriously entertain the possibility that Mr J would be able to describe the bottle as *half-full/half-empty*, and expected that he would therefore be forced back onto syntactic negation. Note that in this situation Mr J did not have to decide which member of the adjective pair was required; what he had to do was negate the structure which was in large measure provided by T. The problem was not a word-finding one now, but one of syntax. What happened was that Mr J showed little ability to meet this problem, in this session; but in the next (number 16) T followed what was to prove a fruitful approach, via those adjectives that permit the possibility of morphological negation. Using pictures of happy and unhappy faces, Mr J was eventually able to produce constructions involving *unhappy* (rather than *sad*); and from this point it was no problem to move to *not happy*. Immediately after this success, Mr J spontaneously started to produce a number of syntactic negatives, including the rather impressive:

'this 'man is nòt so 'tall/

It may well be that this session made contact with incipient structure that was exactly in line with what T was trying to elicit (see p. 179 above). Whatever the case, T continued work on syntactic negation in the next session, in four main steps:

(*i*) First, after revision of *unhappy = not happy*, *unkind = not kind* etc., T concentrated on the same sort of equivalances with new material, where the adjectives are formed with *-ing* (participial adjectives) and are intermediate in status between the class of adjectives proper and the class of verbs (*unwilling = not willing*; *uninteresting = not interesting*; *unamusing = not amusing* etc.). In each case, the *not* Adj form was introduced via the morphologically negated form *un-Adj*.

(*ii*) Then T moved to verbs proper, using the *-ing* form first of all with intransitives (*not running*; *not walking* etc.). Note that here forms in *un-* are not possible.

(*iii*), (*iv*) T subsequently moved to introduce verbs with both a transitive and an intransitive use, such as *eating*, *drinking*, first without the following O, and then with. All proceeded smoothly until the final stage, when certain problems were encountered:

P	'this 'man 'is smòking/	
T	rǐght/	
P	'this 'man 'is nòt 'smoking/	
T	rìght/ thàt's it/	
P	'this 'man 'is nŏt /	
	erm	
	thìs 'man is / smòking a 'pipe/	
T	mhṁ/	
P	thìs 'man is/ .	*confused*

But these were eventually overcome, and syntactic negation was being regularly elicited:

T	'this 'girl is eàting/	
P	'this 'girl is ěating/	
	'this 'girl . 'is . nòt 'eating/	
T	gòod/ thàt's it/	
P	'this 'girl is ěating/	
	'this 'girl is nòt 'eating/	
T	mhṁ/ no 'let's 'put the àpple in/ —	
	'this girl ǐs/ — —	
P	'this 'girl is . 'eating . an ǎpple/	
	'this 'girl is eàting/	
	'this 'girl is eàting/	
T	'this girl is *ī̄n/	
P	*'this 'girl is nòt 'eating/	
	'this 'girl is 'eating an ǎpple/	
T	gŏod/	
P	'this 'girl is nòt 'eating an 'apple/ .	

Conclusion

Of course, we must avoid leaving the impression that we are here reporting on a completed case history. Mr J was still undergoing therapy at the time of writing, and was not then in a position to be discharged. Between April and July, three main areas were worked on:

(*i*)   sequencing and elaboration of structures over the same material
(*ii*) structuring of clause/phrase-level sequences
(*iii*) development of A-elements.

(*i*)   takes up the issue of conjunction; it was noted earlier that Mr J found difficulty in clausal conjunction in structures such as:

thìs 'bus is 'going úp the 'hill/ ánd/ thǐs 'bus is going dòwn the 'hill/

even though the intonation pattern suggested that the desired structure was there in embryo. In an effort to develop clausal conjunction, phrasal conjunction was concentrated on, using elaboration of structures over the same material as is also being used for sequencing tasks. Thus, a picture in a sequence (making up a story) might show a man walking down the street smoking a cigarette; T tried to elicit structures such as:

X is walking (down the street)
X is smoking (a cigarette)

independently at first, and then encouraged Mr J (modelling where necessary) to conjoin them:

X is walking (down the street) and smoking (a cigarette).

A large measure of success was achieved with this technique, and the temporal conjunction *then* was introduced in session 19.

(*ii*) This concerns the problem of linear segmentation, and really represents a new way of trying to tackle it. T used two dimensions systematically in the visual modality, the vertical being used for phrase structure, and the horizontal for clause-level concatenation (using words on cards):

the		
	was	a
fat		
	smoking	cigarette
man		

Eventually, we hoped to get Mr J to perform a 'word-anagram' task (attending to the uses of the two dimensions illustrated here) on this sort of material; but at the time of writing it was too early to say whether this would prove possible, or even if this approach in general would be successful.

(*iii*) Further development of A-elements was required, and for this we tentatively set up the following framework of prepositional types of construction, basing our decisions on the linguistic assumptions described above (pp. 184ff.):

Locative	in/on/near under/beside in front of at the back of	} (the table)
Temporal	in (the holidays) at (Easter) during (this week)	
Causal (including passive agent)	with (the hammer) by (John)	

That is to say, we are assuming, with Lyons (1968, 298–302) and others, that spatial location is basic with regard to these elements, and that temporal and causal functions are progressively more abstract; and that *in* (Locative) is more basic than *at the back of*, *in* (Temporal) more basic than *during* etc. Again, at the time of writing, we were not able to say how successful this approach might be.

However, in spite of the ongoing nature of our work with Mr J, we feel that it is perhaps worth concluding by laying emphasis on three general points. Firstly, concerning the remediation aspect of this approach, we feel confirmed in our belief that developmental norms provide the most reliable scale that we have so far in the notoriously difficult task of deciding on 'grammatical complexity' (see chapter 2). We take it as axiomatic that less complex linguistic constructions and elements should be introduced before more complex ones; and we feel that the best way of implementing this axiom is to take the normal developmental sequence of structures when deciding on order of remediation with the adult dysphasic. We have however noted a number of instances where the remediation procedure differs between adult and child, and this leads on to our second point, which is that we do not wish to be tied to a developmental hypothesis which would require us to believe that adult dysphasics necessarily undergo a language regression which is the mirror-image of the acquisition process (as argued for by Jakobson 1941). We make no claims in this chapter about the order in which syntactic structures come to be lost, either at trauma or in subsequent regression; we are only concerned with the order in which they may be most successfully introduced during remediation. Thirdly, it is important to note the extent to which work with adults requires reference to be made to semantic and sociolinguistic considerations in addition to any basic syntactic analysis. Our comments under this heading, however, are regrettably unsystematic, in comparison with our syntactic procedure—but this, we feel, is symptomatic of the present state of these fields (cf. chapter 1). We can therefore claim little more than pragmatic justification for such notions as 'degree of semantic contrast' used above.

Postscript

We have sought to establish the effectiveness of LARSP as a procedure for assessment and remediation. Before it can be said to be generally applicable, however, two things are necessary. First, we require many more intensive analyses of Ps. The number studied so far is still small, and we would like to extend the number and range of cases. It is important that the analyses be performed by others as well as ourselves, so that we can be sure that there is a system here which is of general applicability across the range of language disorders. Inevitably, modifications will have to be made as LARSP is tried out in different environments and on different populations, and we hope that readers who decide to use this system will keep us informed of their experiences. In particular, we are interested in hearing from people who have modified our approach to suit the needs of restricted types of population, e.g. in deaf or special education, and from those who have developed materials, games, etc. relating to the various grammatical categories recognized, or who have involved parents or relatives in their use.

Secondly, more information about the normative background to LARSP is crucial, to ensure that the assessment and remediation of Ps is based on an account of normal language which is statistically respectable and sociolinguistically informed. These requirements also hold if the gap between individual assessment and the provision of general diagnostic categories is ever to be bridged. As we have seen, group norms of syntactic development and usage are conspicuously absent at present. We hope to go some way towards providing such norms ourselves, by carrying out a standardization study of young children, which would provide us with such information as this:

(*a*) for a representative sample at a given time, profiles of the structures operating at all stages,
(*b*) a comparison of samples at different times,
(*c*) for any particular sample, the proportion of structures represented at a given stage,
(*d*) details about the relationship between the developmental information and the remaining analytic categories on the profile chart.

In the interim, we would be grateful for studies of normal children made in terms of the sampling procedure outlined earlier (chapter 5).

We recommend that readers who would like to see a statistically more fully developed analysis than ours go to Lee 1974. This book appeared too late for us to take detailed account of its findings in relation to our own approach, and our comments about Lee *et al.* in earlier parts of the book are based entirely on her earlier papers. Focussing as they do on points in her approach of which we are critical, it would be misleading to conclude our account without underlining the very great similarities between her approach and ours, which become all the more marked in her book. In such matters as sampling procedure, the drawing up of a developmental chart, and the advice about its use in remedial contexts, the parallelism with our own work is striking and reassuring. The main differences are threefold:

(*a*)   The Lee work involves the use of two procedures, Developmental Sentence Types (DST) and Developmental Sentence Scoring (DSS). DST classifies pre-sentence utterances, indicating areas where grammatical structure is developing; DSS analyses complete sentences. Our approach is a single procedure, which does not make this distinction. Our argument against it would be that the distinction between presentence and sentence is adult-oriented, and impossible to justify theoretically in relation to language acquisition, as Lee herself admits (82); *where's car*, for instance, is considered a complete sentence, but *where car* a pre-sentence (66): this kind of categorization seems to us to be arbitrary, and ignores the very real functional and formal parallels between such pairs of utterances. And in view of the fact that T would often have to combine the two procedures (81), it seems unnecessary and potentially misleading to make a rigid separation between them.

(*b*)   Lee (1974) is an elaboration and modification of the earlier work. The DSS uses the same categories, but is given a weighting reflecting developmental trends more accurately. There has been little change in the categories recognized and scored, however. There is still no real criterial use made of basic sentence-construction types, though Lee allows the importance of this in her introductory account of grammar; exclusion of initial conjunctions is continued (cf. p. 12 above), though Lee admits it is 'unfair' (74); elliptical constructions are still underestimated (85, 117) and classified as incomplete (cf. above p. 13); the sentence point is still kept, though acknowledged to be no more than a gesture towards other grammatical complexity (137); also punctuation continues to be used, instead of intonation (cf. above p. 57).

(*c*)   DSS is scored (but not DST). We remain uncertain of the value of scores when so many complex variables are involved, and prefer an intuitive evaluation of profiles, at least for the time being.

Finally, we are in complete agreement with Lee about the need to keep the grammatical analysis as short as possible (136), and about the need for T to be flexible in its use (cf. pp. 84, 127, 139).

Little attention has been paid here to the use of LARSP solely as a screening procedure. Its effective use for screening on large populations awaits a simplified procedure which cannot be developed until the normative information is available. As the title LARSP suggests, we view the development of a technique for screening as a priority; at present, however, we feel that the provision of specific guidelines would be premature. We would nevertheless welcome accounts from readers who have attempted to implement such a simplified procedure, on the basis of the Syntax Profile.

As long as the ratio of T staff to Ps remains so low, we are aware that many areas of possible application will stay untouched. We therefore strongly support the recommendations of the Quirk Committee on Speech Therapy Services (HMSO 1972) for an increase in therapists, as only with more time can the basic assessment work get done. It is possible that aspects of syntactic analysis might be done by aides, but this is something which as far as we know, has not been discussed. Everyone is aware of the need for a linguistic perspective for T work, but awareness of the time and training it takes to put linguistic knowledge into practice is not so widespread. For our part, we welcome correspondence and recordings concerning particular cases.

Appendix A LARSP Child Data Collection Instructions

Not less than 15 and not more than 30 minutes of taped material should be obtained for each child, ideally as follows:

(*a*) approx. 15 minutes in an unstructured, free play situation (using toys which do not make too much noise); books, pictures etc. should not be used unless you find yourself with no alternative; interviewer should play with the child in what he considers to be a natural, appropriate way; if the child stays fairly quiet, the session can be turned into a prompted dialogue (asking the child what he's doing, what's happening etc.);

(*b*) approx. 15 minutes of dialogue, on some aspect of the child's experience not to do with the immediate play situation.

Exclude the first few minutes of contact with the child from the above times, especially if he is not at ease with the recording situation in some way.

The interviewer should be alone with the child.

As soon after the recording as possible (preferably, *within 24 hours*):

(*i*) Fill out the Recording Data Section below;

(*ii*) Listen through the tape, and write out as much of the child's utterances as you can, concentrating especially on stretches which may cause an outside listener difficulty (e.g. due to immature articulation, family slang), and giving a gloss to those utterances which may not be clear out of context (e.g. *give me that* = give me the toy dog; *fall down* = his lego house has just fallen down; *doggy* = he has just caught sight of his dog);

(*iii*) write your utterances and each of the child's on separate lines, e.g.

    Int. What's that you've got?
    Ch. It's a car.
           Look, it's making a noise.
    Int. Can I have one?
           Have you got one for me? etc.

(*iv*) Fill out the Child Data Sheet.

Recording data sheet

1 Where did the recording take place?
2 Date of recording.
3 Anything abnormal in the child's general behaviour, health etc.?
4 Anything abnormal in the situation, which may have influenced the way he reacted, and which is not obvious from the tape?

Child data sheet

Name:

1 Date of birth: 2 Sex: 3 Age and sex of sibs:
4 Age of father: of mother: 5 Where living now:
6 Occupation of father: of mother:
7 Does either parent have a noticeable regional accent?
8 Have either any obvious speech/hearing impediment?
9 Child's medical history: normal birth?
            any long stays in hospital?
            any major disability/illness?
10 Any school/nursery/creche etc. attendance? (state what kind and how long)
11 Is the child in regular contact with other adults at home? (state relationship)
12 Does the child have any contact with languages other than English? (state which)
13 Give any psychological testing scores which may be available:
14 Any other information you consider relevant:

Appendix B Child Language Assessment Sampling Procedure

Patient: *Sex:*   *Therapist:*

Date of birth: *Place of recording:*

Referred by: *Date and time:*

Reason for referral:

Background information (to be obtained before first session):

1 Date and sex of sibs:

2 Age of father: of mother:

3 Where living now:

4 Father's occupation:

5 Does either parent have a noticeable regional accent? (state which):

6 Is the child in regular contact with other adults at home? (state relationship):

7 Does the child have any contact with languages other than English? (state which):

8 Abnormal social circumstances in family background:

9 Medical history in family (especially details of speech/language/learning disorder among parents or close relatives):

10 P's medical history (including pre- or postnatal, major disabilities or illnesses, periods of hospitalization):

11 Any noteworthy features of developmental history:

12 Assessment results already obtained:
    (*a*) Hearing tests, if any (give date, details of performance):
    (*b*) Language tests, if any (give test used, date and result):
    (*c*) Psychological tests, if any (give test, date and result):

13 School/nursery/creche etc. attendance (state what kind and how long):

14 Details of previous therapy, if any (when, where, by whom, why):

15 Do you have any views about therapeutic procedures to follow in the long term?

During the session

As soon as P has settled, obtain not less than 15 and not more than 30 minutes of taped material, ideally as follows:

(*a*) approx. 15 minutes in an unstructured, free play situation (using toys which do not make too much noise); books, pictures, etc. should not be used unless you find yourself with no alternative; play with the child in what you consider to be a natural, appropriate way; if the child stays fairly quiet, the session can be turned into a prompted dialogue (asking the child what he's doing, what's happening etc.);

(*b*) approx. 15 minutes of dialogue, on some aspect of the child's experience not to do with the immediate play situation.

Exclude the first few minutes of contact with the child from the above times, especially if he is not at ease with the recording situation in some way.

At the end of the session, establish whether it would be possible for P to be taped at home, talking with parent or sib. One or a series of recordings totalling about 10 minutes would suffice.

After the session

1 Listen through the tape, and write out as much of the child's utterance as you can, concentrating especially on stretches which may cause an outside listener difficulty (e.g. due to immature articulation, family slang), and giving a gloss to those utterances which may not be clear out of context (e.g. *give me that* = give me the toy dog; *fall down* = his lego house has just fallen down; *doggy* = he has just caught sight of his dog).

2 Write your utterances and each of the child's on separate lines, e.g.

> T What's that you've got?
> P It's a car.
>   Look, it's making a noise.
> T Can I have one?
>   Have you got one for me? etc.

3 Answer the following questions about the session:

(*a*) Anything noteworthy in the remainder of the session?

(*b*) Were other people present at any stage? (state whom):

(*c*) Rate the session for typicality, as far as you can, in terms of P's normal health, behaviour etc.:

(*d*) Comment on any notable fluctuations in P's behaviour throughout, especially if the variations are not explicable by reference to the tape:

(*e*) Did P react to the tape-recorder at all?

(*f*) Note any linguistic features which struck you as interesting, and to which you think our attention should be drawn:

(*g*) Evaluate the session (e.g. How well do you think it went? How easy did you find it?)

(*h*) Evaluate personal attitudes relating to P. (Do you get on well with him? How does P respond to you? Any noteworthy parental attitudes towards him or his difficulty?)

Next session planned, if any: Date: Venue:

Aims:

Appendix C   Communicative History Form

Name of patient: *Age:*

Address:

What relationship do you have to the patient? (e.g. wife, son, nurse)

Who lives with the patient? (e.g. wife, lives alone, lives in old people's home)

Family:

   Name of wife/husband:

Names of sons	Wife's name	Children's names and ages	Where do they live?
1			
2			
3			

Name of daughters	Husband's name	Children's names and ages	Where do they live?
1			
2			
3			

Names of close relatives (brothers, sisters, in-laws etc.) and any relevant details; only list those whom the patient is likely to mention regularly:

Name	Relationship	Where living?
1		
2		
3		
4		
5		
6		

Names of friends, and any relevant details (e.g. workmates, neighbours):

1

2

3

4

5

6

List any nicknames or special names used in the patient's family which might come up in conversation with us:

Pets:

Give names and type of pet belonging to the patient's family:

Does the patient see any of the above often?

Has anything happened to one of the above recently which might be on the patient's mind?

Have you noticed any change in the attitude of any of the above towards the patient as a result of the illness?

What sort of a person was the patient before the illness (e.g. quiet, talkative, serious, humourous, lively, short-tempered, thoughtful)? Use as many labels as you can think of.

Have you noticed any changes in the patient's behaviour since the illness?

Does the patient express any strong feelings as to *why* his present condition has arisen?

If the patient is physically disabled in any way, as a result of the illness, does he/she express any particularly strong feelings about this?

Is there any particular activity that the patient is no longer able to carry out which causes particular anxiety?

What was the patient's job?

Had he/she retired?

Was the patient ever in the Services? Give details.

Is any work attempted now?

Which sports, teams etc. was the patient interested in, if any?

Did he/she play any sport before the illness?

Name any clubs or societies that the patient belonged to.

Was the patient a churchgoer? Give details.

Television: Programmes and personalities particularly liked and disliked:

Radio: Programmes and personalities particularly liked and disliked:

Music: Is the patient interested in any particular kind of music? Give details.

Does the patient sing, play etc.?

What paper(s) did the patient read regularly before the illness?

Were any magazines read regularly?

Are any of these still read?

Did the patient have any favourite books or authors?

Does he/she wear glasses for reading? (If so, would you please make sure that the patient brings them to therapy sessions.)

Hobbies (e.g. knitting, gardening, films): give details.

Are there any places of particular interest to the patient? (e.g. holiday haunts, week-end visits)

Has the patient ever been abroad? Give details.

Has the patient ever lived anywhere else for a period of time? Give details.

Can you think of anything else we should know about which might stimulate the patient's interest, bring back memories, and generally help to encourage communication?

Can you think of any topics which ought to be avoided, because of their painful associations for the patient?

This form should be returned to the speech therapist.

Note: This form is a synthesis and elaboration of ideas we have seen in use in various clinics: we acknowledge here our thanks to those therapists and teachers who have helped in its construction.

Appendix D Sample of syntactic analysis of adult speech

A　　　　I spotted you in town yesterday, John.
Sentence:　S　V　O　　A　　　A　　Voc
Phrase:　Pron　　　Pron Pr　N
Word:　　　　-ed

B　Where?
S:　　Q
P:
W:

A　　I was in the garage behind the police station, and I saw
S:　　S V　　　　　　　　　A　　　　　　　　c　S　V
P:　Pron　Pr D　N　　Pr　D　Adj　N　　Pron
W:　　-ed　　　　　　　　　　　　　　　　　　　　-ed
　　you　in the market.
S:　　O　　　A
P:　Pron　Pr　D　N
W:

B　　Yes.　We were trying to find some new curtains.
S:　Minor　S　　　V　　　　　　　O
P:　　　　Pron Aux　v　　v　　D　Adj　N
W:　　　　　　-ed　-ing　　　　　　　-pl.
　　But what were you doing in the garage?
S:　c　Q　　　S　V　　　A
P:　　　　Aux Pron　v　Pr D　　N
W:　　　　　-ed　　-ing

A　Looking for a man who could fix my car.
S:　　　V　　　　　　　O
　　　　　　　　　　s　V　　O
P:　　v　part D　N　　Aux　v　D　N
W:　　-ing

I think the back wheel's falling off.

S:	S	V		O			
			S		V		
P:	Pron	D	Adj	N	Aux	v	part
W:			'aux				
			3s			-ing	

B Gosh! Did you succeed?

S:	Minor	S	V
P:		Aux Pron	v
W:		-ed	

A I found a very helpful mechanic, but unfortunately

S:	S	V		O		c	A
P:	Pron	D	Int	Adj	N		
W:		-ed					-ly

he didn't have all the parts.

S:	S	V		O		
P:	Pron	Aux	Neg v	I	D	N
W:			n't			pl.

B That's always the problem.   What a nuisance!

S:	S	V	A	C		Minor
P:	Pron	Cop		D	N	
W:		's				

A. And there's nothing I can do until he gets some from the factory.

S:	and there	V		C			A			
		Cop	Pron	S	V	s	S	V	O	A
P:				Pron	Aux v		Pron	Pron	Pr	D	N
W:		's					3s				

B If I can help in any way, let me know.

S:		A			V_{imp}	O	
	s S	V	A				
P:	Pron Aux v	Pr	D	N	Aux	Pron	v

I shan't be using my car next week, so if you'd like to borrow it,

S:	S	V		O	A	c		A		
P:							s	S	V	O
W:	Aux Neg	Aux	v	D N	Adj N		Pron Aux v		v	Pron
	n't		-ing				'aux			

please do.

S:	A	V_{imp}

A   Thanks very much.   But I think it'll be ready.

S: Minor   c S V   O

                                     S V C

P: Pron   Pron Aux v

W: *'aux*

Glossary of Symbols

		see page
A	adverbial	46
A pos	adverbial position	79
Adj	adjectival	53
Adj seq	adjectival sequence	79
Aux	auxiliary	46
'aux	contracted auxiliary form	55
c	coordinator	47
C	complement	45
Comm	command sentence type	66
conn	connectivity marker	77
cop	copula	45
'cop	contracted copula form	55
D	determiner	53
D	participant in session other than T or P (e.g. doctor, daddy)	139, 142
Det	determiner system (errors)	79
-ed	past tense	54
-en	past participle	54
-er	comparative	55
-est	superlative	55
Excl	exclamatory sentence type	66
FA	forced alternative (question)	120
gen	genitive	55
I	initiator	53
-ing	present participle	54
Int	intensifier	53
let	first person command	72
-ly	adverb marker	55
Mod	modal verb (errors)	79
N	noun	12, 51
'N'	noun-like element at Stage I	64
N Irreg	irregular noun inflections (errors)	79
Neg	negation	54
n't	contracted negative form	54

References

AMIDON, A. and CAREY, P. 1972: Why five-year-olds cannot understand *before* and *after*. *JVLVB* **11**, 417–23.

ANTHONY, A., BOGLE, D., INGRAM, T. T. S. and MCISAAC, M. W. 1971: *The Edinburgh Articulation Test*. Edinburgh and London: Livingstone.

BELLUGI, U. 1965: The development of interrogative structures in children's speech. In K. Riegel (ed.), *The development of language functions*. University of Michigan Language Development Program, Report **8**, 103–38.

BEVINGTON, J. and CRYSTAL, D. 1975: *Skylarks*. London: Nelson.

BLASDELL, R. and JENSEN, P. 1970: Stress and word position as determinants of imitation in first-language learners. *JSHR* **13**, 193–202.

BLOOM, L. M. 1967: A comment on Lee's 'Developmental sentence types: a method for comparing normal and deviant syntactic development'. *JSHD* **32**, 294–6.

— 1970: *Language development: form and function in emerging grammars*. Cambridge, Mass.: MIT Press.

— 1973: *One word at a time: the use of single word utterances before syntax*. The Hague: Mouton.

BRANNON, J. B. and MURRAY, T. 1966: The spoken syntax of normal, hard-of-hearing, and deaf children. *JSHR* **9**, 604–10.

BRAUN, C. and KLASSEN, B. 1971: A transformational analysis of oral syntactic structures of children representing varying ethnolinguistic communities. *Ch. Dev.* **42**, 1859–71.

BROWN, H. D. 1971: Children's comprehension of relativized English sentences. *Ch. Dev.* **42**, 1923–36.

BROWN, R. 1973: *A first language*. Cambridge, Mass.: Harvard University Press.

BROWN, R., CAZDEN, C. and BELLUGI, U. 1969: The child's grammar from I to III. In J. P. Hill (ed.), *Minnesota Symposium on Child Psychology* **2**. Minneapolis: University of Minnesota Press, 28–73.

BROWN, R. and HANLON, C. 1970: Derivational complexity and the order of acquisition in child speech. In Hayes 1970.

CAMBON, J. and SINCLAIR, H. 1974: Relations between syntax and semantics: are they 'easy to see'. *B. J. Psych.* **65**, 133–40.

CAZDEN, C. 1968: The acquisition of noun and verb inflections. *Ch. Dev.* **39**, 433–48.

CHILD, J. P. 1972: A case study. *Bull. Coll. Sp. Th.* **247**, 7–9.

CHOMSKY, C. 1969: *The acquisition of syntax in children from 5 to 10*. Cambridge, Mass.: MIT Press.

CHOMSKY, N. 1957a: *Syntactic structures*. The Hague: Mouton.
— 1957b: Review of B. F. Skinner, *Verbal behavior*. *Lg.* **35**, 26–58.
— 1965: *Aspects of the theory of syntax*. Cambridge, Mass.: MIT Press.
— 1968: *Language and mind*. New York: Harcourt, Brace and World.
— 1970. Deep structure, surface structure and semantic interpretation. In R. Jakobson and S. Kawamoto (eds.), *Studies in general and oriental linguistics*. Tokyo.
CLARK, R., HUTCHESON, S. and VAN BUREN, P. 1974: Comprehension and production in language acquisition. *JL* **10**, 39–54.
CONN, P. 1971: *Remedial syntax*. London: Invalid Children's Aid Association, Occasional Papers **1**.
COOPER, R. L. 1967: The ability of deaf and hearing children to apply phonological rules. *JSHR* **10**, 77–86.
COWAN, P. A., WEBER, J., HADDINOTT, B. A. and KLEIN, J. 1967: Mean length of spoken responses as a function of stimulus, experimenter and subject. *Ch. Dev.* **38**, 191–203.
CROMER, R. F. 1970: Children are nice to understand: surface structure clues for the recovery of a deep structure. *B. J. Psych.* **61**, 397–408.
CRUTTENDEN, A. 1974: An experiment involving comprehension of intonation in children from 7 to 10. *J.Ch.Lang.* **1**, 221–31.
CRYSTAL, D. 1966: English. In *Word classes*, special volume of *Lingua* **17**, 24–56.
— 1969: *Prosodic systems and intonation in English*. London: Cambridge University Press.
— 1971a: *Linguistics*. Harmondsworth, Middx.: Penguin.
— 1971b: Prosodic systems and language acquisition. In P. Léon (ed.), *Prosodic feature analysis*. Montreal: Didier, 77–90.
— 1972a: The case of linguistics: a prognosis. *BJDC* **7**, 3–16.
— 1972b: Syntax matters. In *Proceedings of 1972 National Conference of Teachers of the Deaf*.
— 1973a: Nonsegmental phonology in language acquisition: a review of the issues. *Lingua* **32**, 1–45.
— 1973b: *Basic linguistics* and *Language acquisition*. Cassette tapes and slides. Reading University: Reading Centre.
— 1974a: Neglected linguistic principles in the study of reading. In UKRA *Proceedings of 11th Annual Study Congress*.
— 1974b: Review of R. Brown, *A first language J.Ch.Lang.* **1**, 289–307.
CRYSTAL, D. and CRAIG, E. (in press): Contrived sign language. In I. Schlesinger and L. Namir (eds.), *Current trends in the study of sign language of the deaf.*
CRYSTAL, D. and DAVY, D. 1969: *Investigating English style*. London: Longman.
— 1975: *Advanced conversational English*. London: Longman.
DALE, P. S. 1972: *Language development: structure and function*. Hinsdale, Ill.: Dryden Press.
DARLEY, F. and MOLL, K. 1960: Reliability of language measures and sizes of language sample. *JSHR* **3**, 166–73.
DAVIS, E. A. 1938: Developmental changes in the distribution of parts of speech. *Ch. Dev.* **9**, 309–17.

DAVIS, G. A. 1973: Linguistics and language therapy: the language construction board. *JSHD* **38**, 205–14.

DEPARTMENT OF EDUCATION AND SCIENCE. 1972: *Speech therapy services*. London: HMSO.

DERWING, B. L. 1973: *Transformational grammar as a theory of language acquisition*. London: Cambridge University Press.

DEVER, R. B. 1972a: *TALK (Teaching the American Language to Kids)*. Experimental Materials. Final Report **27.3**. Bloomington, Indiana University: Center for Innovation in Teaching the Handicapped.

— 1972b: A comparison of the results of a revised version of Berko's test of morphology with the free speech of mentally retarded children. *JSHA* **15**, 169–78.

—1973: The development of the clause: toward a unified theory of language development in children. Mimeo.

DEVER, R. B. and BAUMAN, P. M. 1971: Scale of children's clausal development. Mimeo. Reprinted in Longhurst 1974.

DEVER, R. B. and GARDNER, W. 1971: Performance of normals and retardates on Berko's test of morphology. *Lg. and Sp.* **13**, 162–81.

DONALDSON, M. C. and WALES, R. J. 1970: On the acquisition of some relational terms. In Hayes 1970, 235–68.

DORE, J. 1975: Holophrases, speech acts and language universals. *J.Ch.Lg.* **2**, 21–40.

EISENSON, J. and INGRAM, D. 1972: Childhood aphasia – an updated concept based on recent research. *Acta Symbolica* **3**, 108–16.

ELLSWORTH, R. B. 1951: The repression of schizophrenic language. *J.Consult. Psychol.* **15**, 387–91.

ELSON, B. and PICKETT, V. 1965: *An introduction to morphology and syntax*. Santa Ana, Calif.: SIL.

ENGLER, L. F., HANNAH, E. P. and LONGHURST, T. M. 1973: Linguistic analysis of speech samples: a practical guide for clinicians. *JSHD* **38**, 192–204.

FERGUSON, C. A. and SLOBIN, D. I. (eds.) 1973: *Studies of child language development*. New York: Holt, Rinehart and Winston.

FILLENBAUM, S., JONES, L. V. and WEPMAN, J. M. 1961: Some linguistic features of speech from aphasic patients. *Lg. and Sp.* **4**, 91–108.

FODOR, J. and GARRETT, M. 1966: Some reflections on competence and performance. In Lyons and Wales 1966, 135–62.

FOSTER, C. R., GIDDAN, J. J. and STARK, J. (n.d.): *ACLC: Assessment of Children's Language Comprehension*. Palo Alto: Consulting Psychologists Press.

FRASER, G. M. and BLOCKLEY, J. 1973: *The language-disordered child*. Slough, Bucks.: NFER.

FYGETAKIS, L. J. and INGRAM, D. 1972: Language rehabilitation and programmed conditioning: a case study. *PRCLD* **4**, 169–78.

GIMSON, A. C. 1970: *An introduction to the pronunciation of English*, 2nd edn. London: Edward Arnold.

GLEASON, J. B. 1973: Code switching in children's language. In Moore 1973, 159–67.

GODA, S. 1964: Spoken syntax of normal, deaf, and retarded adolescents. *JVLVB* **3**, 401–5.

GOODGLASS, H. 1968: Studies on the grammar of aphasics. In S. Rosenberg and J. Koplin (eds.), *Developments in applied psycholinguistics research*. New York: Macmillan, 177–208.

GOODGLASS, H., FODOR, I. G. and SCHULHOFF, C. 1967: Prosodic factors in grammar – evidence from aphasia. *JSHR* **10**, 5–20.

GOODGLASS, H. and HUNT, J. 1958: Grammatical complexity and aphasic speech. *Word* **14**, 197–207.

GOTTSLEBEN, R. H., TYACK, D. and BUSCHINI, G. 1974: Three case studies in language training: applied linguistics. *JSHD* **39**, 213–23.

GRAHAM, J. T. and GRAHAM, L. W. 1971: Language behavior of the mentally retarded: syntactic characteristics. *A.J.Ment.Def.* **75**, 623–9.

GREENFIELD, P., SMITH, J. and LAUFER, P. (in press): *Communication and the beginnings of language: the development of semantic structure in one-word speech and beyond*. New York: Academic Press.

GRIFFITH, J. and MINER, L. E. 1969: LCI reliability and size of language sample. *J. Comm. Dis.* **2**, 264–7.

HAHN, E. 1948: Analyses of the content and form of the speech of first-grade children. *Q.J.Sp.* **34**, 361–6.

HART, B. 1975: The use of adult cues to test the language competence of young children. *J.Ch.Lang.* **2**, 105–24.

HASS, W. A. and WEPMAN, J. M. 1969: Surface structure, deep structure, and transformations: a model for syntactic development. *JSHD* **34**, 303–11.

HATFIELD, F. M. 1972: Looking for help from linguistics. *BJDC* **7**, 64–81.

HAYES, J. R. (ed.) 1970: *Cognition and the development of language*. New York: Wiley.

HEIDER, F. R. and HEIDER, G. M. 1940: A comparison of sentence structure of deaf and hearing children. *Psychol. Monog.* **52**, 42–103.

HERRIOT, P. 1969: The comprehension of tense by young children. *Ch. Dev.* **40**, 103–10.

HOCKETT, C. F. 1958: *A course in modern linguistics*. New York: Macmillan.

HOCKETT, C. F. and ALTMANN, S. A. 1968: A note on design features. In T. A. Sebeok (ed.), *Animal communication*. Bloomington: Indiana University Press, 61–72.

HOWES, D. 1967: Some experimental investigations of language in aphasia. In K. Salzinger and S. Salzinger (eds.), *Research in verbal behavior and some neurophysiological implications*. New York: Academic Press, 181–96.

HUNT, K. 1964: *Differences in grammatical structures written at three grade levels, the structures to be analysed by transformational methods*. Report to US Office of Education, Cooperative Research Project **1998**. Tallahassee, Florida.

— 1970: Syntactic maturity in schoolchildren and adults. *Monogr. Soc. Res. Ch. Dev.* **35**.

HUTCHINSON, M. K. F. 1972: An experiment in applying linguistics to speech therapy. *BJDC* **7**, 49–53.

HUTTENLOCHER, J. 1974: The origins of language comprehension. In R. L. Solso (ed.), *Theories in cognitive psychology: the Loyola Symposium.* New York: Wiley.

HUXLEY, R. 1970: The development of the correct use of subject personal pronouns in two children. In G. B. Flores d'Arcais and W. J. M. Levelt (eds.), *Advances in psycholinguistics.* London: North-Holland, 141–65.

INGRAM, D. 1972a: The acquisition of the English verbal auxiliary and copula in normal and linguistically deviant children. *PRCLD* **4**, 79–91.

— 1972b: Language program for linguistically deviant children. Stanford University, School of Medicine, unpublished.

— 1972c: The development of phrase-structure rules. *Lang. Learning* **22**, 65–77.

— 1972d: The acquisition of questions and its relation to cognitive development in normal and linguistically deviant children: a pilot study. *PRCLD* **4**, 13–18.

JESPERSEN, O. 1922: *Language: its nature, development, and origin.* London: Allen and Unwin.

JOHNSON, W., DARLEY, F. L. and SPRIESTERSBACH, D. C. 1963: *Diagnostic methods in speech pathology.* New York: Harper and Row.

JONES, L. V. and WEPMAN, J. M. 1967: Grammatical indicants of speaking style in normal and aphasic speakers. In K. Salzinger and S. Salzinger (eds.), *Research in verbal behavior and some neurophysiological implications.* New York: Academic Press, 169–80.

JONES, L. V., GOODMAN, M. F. and WEPMAN, J. M. 1963: The classification of parts of speech for the characterization of aphasia. *Lg. and Sp.* **6**, 94–108.

JOOS, M. (ed.) 1957: *Readings in linguistics* I. London: University of Chicago Press.

JORDAN, C. M. and ROBINSON, W. P. 1972: The grammar of working and middle-class children using elicited imitations. *Lg. and Sp.* **15**, 122–40.

KEENEY, T. J. and WOLFE, J. 1972: The acquisition of agreement in English. *JVLVB* **11**, 698–705.

KIRK, S. A. 1966: The diagnosis and remediation of psycholinguistic disabilities. University of Illinois: Institute for Research on Exceptional Children.

KIRK, S. A. and KIRK, W. D. 1971: *Psycholinguistic learning disabilities: diagnosis and remediation.* Chicago: University of Illinois Press.

KIRK, S. A., MCCARTHY, J. and KIRK, W. D. 1968: *The Illinois Test of Psycholinguistic Abilities.* Urbana: University of Illinois Press.

KLIMA, E. S. and BELLUGI, U. 1966: Syntactic regularities in the speech of children. In Lyons and Wales, 1966.

LACKNER, J. 1968: A developmental study of language behavior in retarded children. *Neuropsychol.* **6**, 301–20.

LEE, L. 1966: Developmental sentence types. *JSHD* **31**, 311–30.

— 1969: *The Northwestern Syntax Screening Test.* Evanston, Ill.: Northwestern University.

— 1974: *Developmental sentence analysis: a grammatical assessment procedure for speech and language disorders.* Evanston, Ill.: Northwestern University.

LEE, L. and CANTER, S. M. 1971: Developmental sentence scoring: a clinical procedure for estimating syntactic development in children's spontaneous speech. *JSHD* **36**, 315–40.

LEE, L., KOENIGSKNECHT, R. A. and MULHERN, S. T. 1975: *Interactive language development teaching: the clinical presentation of grammatical structure.* Evanston, Ill.: Northwestern University.

LENNEBERG, E. H. 1967: *Biological foundations of language.* New York: Wiley.

LENNEBERG, E. H., NICHOLS, I. A. and ROSENBERGER, E. F. 1964: Primitive stages of language development in mongolism. In *Disorders of Communication* **42**: *Research Publications.* Baltimore, Maryland: Williams and Wilkins.

LEONARD, L. B. 1972: What is deviant language? *JSHD* **37**, 427–46.

LEREA, L. 1958: Assessing language development. *JSHR* **1**, 75–85.

LIMBER, J. 1973: The genesis of complex sentences. In Moore 1973, 169–85.

LONGHURST, T. M. (ed.) 1974: *Linguistic analysis of children's speech: readings.* New York: MSS Information Corporation.

LONGHURST, T. M. and SCHRANDT, T. A. M. 1973: Linguistic analysis of children's speech: a comparison of four procedures. *JSHD* **38**, 240–49.

LOZAR, B., WEPMAN, J. M. and HASS, W. 1973: Syntactic indices of language use of mentally retarded and normal children. *Lg. and Sp.* **16**, 22–33.

LYONS, J. 1963: *Structural semantics.* Publications of the Philological Society **20**. Oxford: Basil Blackwell.

— 1968: *Introduction to theoretical linguistics.* London: Cambridge University Press.

— 1970: *Chomsky.* London: Fontana.

— 1973: Human language. In R. A. Hinde (ed.), *Nonverbal communication.* London: Cambridge University Press, 49–85.

LYONS, J. and WALES, R. (eds.) 1966: *Psycholinguistics papers.* Edinburgh University Press.

MACDONALD, J. D. and NICKOLS, M. 1974: *Environmental language inventory:* a *semantic-based assessment for training generalized communication.* Ohio State University: The Nisonger Center.

MACKAY, D. D., THOMPSON, B. and SCHAUB, I. 1970: *Breakthrough to literacy.* Teacher's Manual. London: Longman.

MACKEY, W. F. 1965: *Language teaching analysis.* London: Longman.

MATTHEWS, P. H. 1974: *Inflectional morphology.* London: Cambridge University Press.

MCCARTHY, D. 1930: *The language development of the pre-school child.* Minneapolis: University of Minnesota.

— 1954. Language development in children. In L. Carmichael (ed.), *Manual of child psychology.* New York: Wiley, 492–630.

MCCAWLEY, J. D. 1968: The role of semantics in a grammar. In E. Bach and R. Harms (eds.), *Universals in linguistic theory.* New York: Holt, Rinehart and Winston.

MCGRATH, C. O. and KUNZE, L. H. 1973: Development of phrase structure rules involved in tag questions elicited from children. *JSHR* **16**, 498–512.

MCNEILL, D. 1966: Developmental psycholinguistics. In F. Smith and G. A. Miller (eds.), *The genesis of language.* Cambridge, Mass.: MIT Press, 15–84.

— 1970: *The acquisition of language.* New York: Harper and Row.

MENYUK, P. 1963: Syntactic structures in the language of children. *Ch. Dev.* **34**, 407–22.

— 1964: Comparison of grammar of children with functionally deviant and normal speech. *JSHR* **7**, 109–21.

— 1969: *Sentences children use.* Cambridge, Mass.: MIT Press.

— 1971: *The acquisition and development of language.* Englewood Cliffs: Prentice-Hall.

MENYUK, P. and LOONEY, P. L. 1972: A problem of language disorder: length versus structure. *JSHR* **15**, 264–79.

MILLER, J. F. 1973: Sentence imitation in preschool children. *Lg. and Sp.* **16**, 1–14.

MILLER, J. F. and YODER, D. 1974: Teaching language to retardates. In R. L. Schiefelbusch and L. L. Lloyd (eds.), *Language perspectives — acquisition, retardation and intervention.* Baltimore, Maryland: University Park Press.

MINER, L. E. 1969: Scoring procedures for the length-complexity index: a preliminary report. *J. Comm. Dis.* **2**, 224–40.

MINIFIE, F., DARLEY, F. and SHERMAN, D. 1963: Temporal reliability of seven language measures. *JSHR* **6**, 139–48.

MITTLER, P., JEFFREE, D., WHELDALL, K. and BERRY, P. 1974: *Assessment and remediation of language comprehension and production in severely subnormal children.* University of Manchester: Hester Adrian Research Centre.

MOORE, T. E. 1973: *Cognitive development and the acquisition of language.* New York: Academic Press.

MOREHEAD, D. M. 1972: Early grammatical and semantic relations: some implications for a general representational deficit in linguistically deviant children. *PRCLD* **4**, 1–12.

MOREHEAD, D. M. and INGRAM, D. 1973: The development of base syntax in normal and linguistically deviant children. *JSHR* **16**, 330–52.

MOREHEAD, D. M. and JOHNSON, M. 1972: Piaget's theory of intelligence applied to the assessment and treatment of linguistically deviant children. *PRCLD* **4**, 143–61.

MORLEY, H. J. 1960: Applying linguistics to speech and language therapy for aphasics. *Lang. Learn.* **10**, 135–49.

MUMA, J. R. 1971: Syntax of preschool fluent and disfluent speech: a transformational analysis. *JSHR* **14**, 428–41.

— 1973a: Language assessment: the Co-occurring and Restricted Structure procedure (CORS). *Acta Symbolica* **4**, 12–29.

— 1973b: Language assessment: some underlying assumptions. *ASHA* **15**, 331–8.

MYERSON, R. and GOODGLASS, H. 1972: Transformational grammars of aphasic patients. *Lg. and Sp.* **15**, 40–50.

MYKLEBUST, H. 1965: *Development and disorders of written language.* New York: Grune and Stratton.

NELSON, K. E., CARSKADDON, G. and BONVILLIAN, J. D. 1973: Syntax acquisition: impact of experimental variation in adult verbal interaction with the child. *Ch. Dev.* **44**, 497–504.

NEWFIELD, M. U. and SCHLANGER, B. B. 1968: The acquisition of English morphology by normal and educable mentally retarded children. *JSHR* **11**, 693–706.

NICE, M. M. 1925: Length of sentences as a criterion of a child's progress in speech. *J. Educ. Psych.* **16**, 370–79.

O'CONNOR, J. D. 1973: *Phonetics*. Harmondsworth, Middx: Penguin.

O'DONNELL, R., GRIFFIN, W. and NORRIS, R. 1967: *Syntax of kindergarten and elementary schoolchildren: a transformational analysis. NCTE* **8**.

PIAGET, J. 1952: *The origins of intelligence in children*. New York: Norton.

— 1970: Piaget's theory. In P. H. Mussen (ed.), *Carmichael's manual of child psychology* **1**, New York: Wiley.

PRESSNELL, L. M. 1973: Hearing-impaired children's comprehension and production of syntax in oral language. *JSHR* **16**, 12–21.

QUIRK, R., GREENBAUM, S., LEECH, G. and SVARTVIK, J. 1972: *A grammar of contemporary English*. London: Longman.

QUIRK, R. and GREENBAUM, S. 1973. *A university grammar of English*. London: Longman.

QUIRK, R. and SVARTVIK, J. 1966: *Investigating linguistic acceptability*. The Hague: Mouton.

REES, N. S. 1971: Bases of decision in language training. *JSHD* **36**, 283–304.

— 1973: Auditory processing factors in language disorders: the view from Procrustes' bed. *JSHD* **38**, 304–15.

REID, J. and LOW, J. 1973: *Link-up*. Edinburgh: Holmes McDougall.

RENFREW, C. (n.d.): *The bus story*. Published by the author.

REYNELL, J. 1969: *Developmental language scale*. Slough, Bucks.: NFER.

ROBINS, R. 1971: *General linguistics: an introductory survey*, 2nd edn. London: Longman.

RODD, L. J. and BRAINE, M. D. S. 1970: Children's imitations of syntactic constructions as a measure of linguistic competence. *JVLVB* **10**, 430–43.

ROSENBAUM, P. S. 1967: Specification and utilization of a transformational grammar. In Project Report **4641**, IBM Watson Research Center.

ROSENBERG, S. 1973: Problems of language development in children: a discussion of Olson's review. In H. C. Haywood (ed.), *Sociocultural aspects of mental retardation*. New York: Appleton Century Crofts.

ROSENTHAL, W. S., EISENSON, J. and LUCKAU, J. M. 1972: A statistical test of the validity of diagnostic categories used in childhood language disorders: implications for assessment procedures. *PRCLD* **4**, 121–41.

SCHNEIDERMAN, N. 1955: A study of the relationship between articulatory disability and language ability. *JSHD* **20**, 359–64.

SCHUELL, H. 1965: *The Minnesota test for differential diagnosis of aphasia: administrative manual and card materials*. Minneapolis: University of Minnesota Press.

SEFER, J. W. and SHAW, R. 1972: The use of psycholinguistic principles in the treatment of aphasia. *BJDC* **7**, 87–9.

SHARF, D. J. 1972: Some relationships between measures of early language development. *JSHD* **37**, 64–74.

SHERMAN, D., SHRINER, T. H. and SILVERMAN, F. 1965: Psychological scaling of language development of children. *Proc. Iowa Acad. Sc.* **72**, 366–71.

SHIPLEY, E. F., SMITH, C. S. and GLEITMAN, L. R. 1969: A study in the acquisition of language. *Lg.* **45**, 322–42.

SHRINER, T. H. 1967: A comparison of selected measures with psychological scale values of language development. *JSHR* **10**, 828–35.

— 1969: A review of mean length of response as a measure of expressive language development in children. *JSHD* **34**, 61–8.

SHRINER, T. H. and MINER, L. 1968: Morphological structures in the language of disadvantaged and advantaged children. *JSHR* **11**, 605–10.

SHRINER, T. H. and SHERMAN, D. 1967: An equation for assessing language development. *JSHR* **10**, 41–8.

SHULTZ, T. R. and PILON, R. 1973: Development of the ability to detect linguistic ambiguity. *Ch. Dev.* **44**, 728–33.

SINCLAIR-DE-ZWART, H. 1969: Developmental psychological linguistics. In D. Elkind and J. Flavell (eds.), *Studies in cognitive development.* London: Oxford University Press.

SLOBIN, D. I. and WELSH, C. A. 1968: Elicited imitation as a research tool in developmental psycholinguistics. Working Paper **10**, Language Behavior Research Laboratory, Berkeley. Reprinted in C. A. Ferguson and D. I. Slobin (eds.) 1973, *Studies in child language development.* New York: Harper and Row, 485–97.

SMITH, M. 1933: The influence of age, sex, and situation on the frequency, form, and function of questions asked by preschool children. *Ch. Dev.* **4**, 201–13.

SPREEN, O. and WACHAL, R. S. 1973: Psycholinguistic analysis of aphasic language: theoretical formulations and procedures. *Lg. and Sp.* **16**, 130–46.

STACK, E. M. 1971: *The language laboratory and modern language teaching.* London: Oxford University Press.

STARK, J., POPPEN, R. and MAY, M. Z. 1967: Effects of alterations of prosodic features on the sequencing performance of aphasic children. *JSHR* **10**, 844–48.

STOKOE, W. 1972: *Semiotics and human sign language.* The Hague: Mouton.

STRAUSS, A. A. and MCCARUS, E. N. 1953: A. linguist looks at aphasia in children. *JSHD* **23**, 54–8.

SVARTVIK, J. (ed.), 1973: *Errata—papers in error analysis.* Lund: Gleerup.

TAYLOR, O. L. and ANDERSON, C. B. 1968: Neuropsycholinguistics and language retraining. In J. W. Black and E. G. Jancosek (eds.), *Proc. Conf. on Language Retraining for Aphasics.* Ohio State University, 3–18.

TEMPLIN, M. 1957: *Certain language skills in children.* Minneapolis: University of Minnesota Press.

THOMAS, F. J. 1971: *Guidelines.* English language course, Stage 1. Woodford Green, Essex: Woodford Educational Publications.

TRUDGILL, P. 1974: *Sociolinguistics.* Harmondsworth, Middx.: Penguin.

TYACK, D. 1972a: The use of language samples in clinical settings. *PRCLD* **4**, 163–8.

— 1972b: Some notes on Lee and Canter's 'Developmental sentence scoring: a clinical procedure for estimating syntactic development in children's spontaneous speech'. *PRCLD* **4**, 179–84.

WACHAL, R. S. and SPREEN, O. 1970: Grammatical analysis of aphasic language. Manual of instructions for classification and coding. University of Victoria. Mimeo.

— 1973: Some measures of lexical diversity in aphasic and normal language performance, *Lg. and Sp.* **16**, 169–81.

WEBSTER, B. and INGRAM, D. 1972: The comprehension and production of the anaphoric pronouns 'he, she, him, her' in normal and linguistically deviant children. *PRCLD* **4**, 55–77.

WEIGL, E. and BIERWISCH, M. 1970: Neuropsychology and linguistics: topics of common research. *FL* **6**, 1–18.

WEPMAN, J. M. and HASS, W. A. 1967: Lexical and syntactic indices of children's language development. In *Actes du Xème Congrès des Linguistes*. Bucharest: Editions de l'Académie de la République Socialiste de Roumanie.

WEPMAN, J. M. and JONES, L. V. 1964: Five aphasias: a commentary on aphasia as a regressive linguistic phenomenon. In D. M. Rioch and E. A. Weinstein (eds.), *Disorders of communication*. Baltimore, Maryland.

WEST, J. J. and WEBER, J. L. 1974: A linguistic analysis of the morphemic and syntactic structures of a hard-of-hearing child. *Lg. and Sp.* **17**, 68–79.

WILLIAMS, F. and NAREMORE, R. C. 1969: Social class differences in children's syntactic performance: a quantitative analysis of field study data. *JSHD* **34**, 779–93.

WILSON, M. E. 1969: A standardized method for obtaining a spoken language sample. *JSHR* **12**, 95–102.

YNGVE, V. 1960: A model and an hypothesis for language structure. *Proc. A. Phil. Soc.* **108**, 275–81.

Index (names)

Index (subjects)